CW00765418

Breaking
the Heart
Open

Breaking the Heart Open

The Shaping of a Psychologist

TONY BATES

Gill Books

Gill Books
Hume Avenue
Park West
Dublin 12
www.gillbooks.ie

Gill Books is an imprint of M.H. Gill and Co.

Design and print origination by O'K Graphic Design, Dublin
Edited by Kerri Ward
Proofread by Liza Costello
Printed and bound in Great Britain by Clays Ltd, Elcograf S.p.A.
This book is typeset in 11/18 pt Minion Pro.

This book is intended as general guidance only and does not in any way represent medical advice for individual persons. Readers are advised to attend their own healthcare professionals for advice and guidance appropriate to their particular needs. This book does not in any way replace the advice and guidance that your own doctor or other healthcare professional can give you. If you are concerned about any of the issues raised in this book, be sure to consult your doctor.
Archival case histories have been anonymised.

The paper used in this book comes from the wood pulp of sustainably managed forests.

For permission to reproduce text, the author and publisher gratefully acknowledge the following:
© *The Irish Times*
© Macmillan Children's Books

A CIP catalogue record for this book is available from the British Library.
5 4 3 2 1

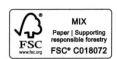

To Ursula, Andrew, Philip and Rachel, with love.

CONTENTS

Vulnerability is the very thing that permits us to connect with each other and recognise in others the same discomfort we have in ourselves. Vulnerability is the engine of compassion and can be a superpower, a special vision that allows us to see the quivering, wounded inner world that most of us possess.

NICK CAVE

INTRODUCTION

Our wounds and how we deal with them shape who we become. For most of my early life, I survived by hiding. I was a 'good' boy and did my best to fit in and be 'normal', but beneath this charade, I mostly felt terrified and alone. I experienced the world as a place where bad things could happen, even if I couldn't explain what it was that frightened me. I was ashamed of how badly I felt and worried that if other people knew, they would be disappointed that I wasn't the easy-going person I pretended to be.

Being quiet, compliant and slightly withdrawn made me a perfect target for bullies. I was terrified of conflict and surrendered immediately to their taunts, passively taking whatever was doled out. My friends always seemed more 'together' than I was; they knew stuff, they were confident and they had more fun than I did. I was always careful to hide my insecurities in case they might turn against me. I wasn't much fun to be around.

I pushed denial and repression to their limits but always felt uneasy inside. Something wasn't right. That 'something' was probably not one thing, but it felt like a basic wound in my psyche that kept reopening and pulling me under. As I grew up, this wound became inflamed in situations that should have been some of the happiest moments in my life. I longed to fall in love and be loved, but I found intimacy extremely painful. My demons were at their worst in the arms of someone I loved. My insecurities took the form of massive separation anxiety and irrational jealousy.

Life took me out of myself in my twenties. My focus shifted to finishing college, finding a job, getting married, acquiring a home and starting a family. I had 'mini-breakdowns' along the way, but I saved the big one until my thirties. Perhaps I needed to reach a point where I felt strong and safe enough to fall apart. Or perhaps the pain had to get stronger for me to recognise that I'd become a stranger to myself.

'All our sorrows can be borne if you can put them into a story', wrote the author Isak Dinesen. Mental health is a story that can be told, a story that is robust enough to hold our pain. We struggle to a greater or lesser extent with 'unstoried' experiences – body sensations, emotions and memory fragments – for which we haven't yet found a way to express and come to terms with.

In his play *Translations*, Brian Friel, the Irish dramatist, captured this tension we can feel when the story we tell ourselves doesn't do justice to the complexity of our lives. He wrote, 'It can happen that a civilisation can be imprisoned in a linguistic contour which no longer matches the landscape of experience.' The stories we tell ourselves about who we are can either stifle or free us. When they fit what we are experiencing, make sense of how we feel in terms of our past and present struggles, they help us to feel real and bear the unbearable. But when they are superficial or simplistic and don't match our experience, we feel at odds with ourselves. We can't make sense of what we feel. We wonder if there is something terribly wrong with us.

I lived inside a story that was too small for years. I tried to live up to an ideal image of myself – intelligent, socially aware – that never fitted with all I felt inside. Doubts, insecurities and spasms of fear swept through my inner world. My identity didn't fit the shape of my soul. I needed a more robust story that matched the 'landscape of my experience'. A story that allowed me to be more real and gave me room to grow.

This book is about what happened when I came out of hiding and allowed my mind and body to heal slowly. It is for everyone who carries deeper wounds that seem to shadow their every step and that become easily inflamed. It is the story of what I learned from my own pain and the pain of the people I served.

I spent most of my career working in a city centre psychiatric hospital. The people I worked with bore the scars of very difficult lives. Many had struggled to keep their wounds hidden until they reached a breaking point where they could no longer do so. Their vulnerability created an opportunity for honest conversations that didn't routinely happen in the 'normal' world. Some had become embittered by their pain, but most struggled to find relief, to find themselves.

They accepted support despite believing for years that they had to go it alone. Together we faced their fear and bewilderment, sadness and rage. We gave what had been hidden or disowned room to breathe. We knitted fragments of emotions and memory into a coherent story. We learned to appreciate unusual ideas, intense feelings and behaviours that initially made no sense, but which were their best attempt to survive a difficult situation.

Recovery takes time. It always takes longer than the books say to recover a sense of Self. Some people find this tedious. It can be demoralising to circle back over old wounds that still become inflamed despite best efforts at acceptance and self-care. There are periods of painful uncertainty where a person might not know whether they are making progress or falling back. But working in psychology has taught me that pain is the door we walk through to find ourselves. We can try to repress, numb and project it onto others, but we will never be comfortable in our skin until we can recognise it, be with it and give it a place in the larger story of our lives.

Sometimes we haven't been allowed to voice our vulnerabilities because to do so would risk rejection, exclusion or worse. Something can remain unsayable because it's never been spoken about in this family, this community or this society. As we move out into the world, the pain that was unsayable lives on in our bodies. It breaks out in physical symptoms and harmful behaviour patterns. We find this confusing if we live with it or see it around us. In sheer desperation, a young person may choose to calm their body through drugs, drinking, self-harm and a host of other possibilities, seeking a way to stop what isn't working in their body. Or they may choose to end their life.

It's easy to make mental health sound like a completely personal issue; a matter for each of us, alone, to resolve. This is not an accurate or helpful way to look at our lives. Our relationships and social circumstances profoundly shape how we feel about ourselves and manage our lives.

We talk about our emotional struggles more openly today. 'We all have mental health' is our new mantra. It has replaced the fear and shame of my mother's generation who lived by the creed, 'Not a word'. The stigma surrounding mental health difficulties has been reduced, mainly due to service users speaking openly about their experiences. They have shown us that recovery is possible and told us what helps and what doesn't help.

But one of the unintended consequences of our anti-stigma campaigns is that we are increasingly medicalising our problems by framing them in the language of diagnostic psychiatry. There is a growing tendency to see feelings of loneliness, self-doubt, sadness, anxiety and frustration as indicative of something 'wrong'. The complexity and subtlety of our emotional problems may be reduced to a 'chemical imbalance', 'brain anomaly' or 'faulty genes'. No conclusive evidence supports this way of thinking about human distress, but we continue to use labels as if they alone can explain our pain and confusion. We need more robust stories about our mental health that make sense of our wounds and scars and allow us to come to terms with them.

Just as physical pain draws attention to what is hurting in our bodies, our troubled emotions are also messengers. They point to something in our lives that needs our attention and care. Rather than dismiss emotional pain as a biological malfunction, or a disease, we need to respect that our symptoms may reflect some unresolved issues in our past or some oppressive life situation in our present.

Young people are accumulating psychiatric labels at an increasing rate. Access to vital resources may insist that a child first has a diagnosis. A school principal I spoke to recently told me about a student of 17 who announced to her with apparent relief: 'I know what's wrong with me, I have borderline personality disorder.' It was true that she felt unstable, but it was also true that this girl was emotionally exhausted from trying to appease her parents, who were constantly fighting with each other.

Another consequence of framing children's mental health problems purely as 'mental illness' is that psychotropic drug prescriptions have risen exponentially over the past 10 years. A pharmacist shared with me that what she found most 'hurtful' in her work is filling prescriptions of psychiatric medication for children as young as eight. She saw parents as having lost all confidence in themselves to handle their child's distress and was frustrated by our collective refusal to admit how stressful family life has become (for everyone), and the limited latitude there is for children who don't fit neatly into performance-oriented school regimes.

Wonderful front-line mental health workers and highly compassionate clinicians exist. And there are pockets of creative innovation that engage troubled people in dignified and effective ways. But a curious malaise hangs over our mental health service. Perhaps this is a result of our collective failure to give distressed people and their families the support they need. Despite sizeable annual increases in funding and ambitious mental health policies, something is not working. Mental health workers themselves lose heart as they watch familiar faces staying longer in services and taking increasing amounts of drugs for extended periods of time. Service users feel short-changed, workers feel frustrated, and accessing support grows increasingly difficult. The system tasked with supporting those of us who become depressed is, itself, depressed.

In her book, *Strangers to Ourselves*, Rachel Aviv, who was hospitalised at six years old and diagnosed with anorexia, wrote:

> Mental illnesses are often seen as chronic and intractable forces that can take over our lives, but I wonder how much the stories we tell about them, especially in the

beginning, can shape their course. People can feel freed by these stories, but they can also get stuck in them.[1]

My work has exposed me to writers and teachers whose insights into emotional suffering are full of humanity and wisdom. But nothing has shaped the psychologist I've become more than those who allowed me into the dark corners of their lives. They showed me the terror and the beauty of being human. Their recovery always brought them closer to their humanity. And they invited me, in turn, to deepen my own.

Relationships and language hold us together. We can help each other create stories that fit 'the landscape of our experience'. Stories that are as rich and layered as our lives. Stories that are flexible enough to grow as we grow. This book is my story. It traces experiences that profoundly shaped the psychologist I became.

'People can become trapped in history, and history becomes trapped in us', wrote James Baldwin. But when we can face and understand our personal and collective uneasiness, we discover that history does not have to become our destiny.

PROLOGUE

IN THE END IS MY BEGINNING

When the nurse called to say they were moving her to the hospice, I knew something had changed. She had been diagnosed with a brain tumour a month after her 90th birthday but seemed fine. We'd been busy since putting the necessary supports in place to allow her to return home and live out whatever time she had as peacefully as possible.

But Mum's sudden transfer from the general hospital suggested that mightn't happen. I drove to the hospice and arrived as she was settling in. Her room was far more spacious than anything we had at home. No medical paraphernalia surrounded her bed, as there had been in the general hospital.

When I bent over to hug her, she was smiling. One of her eyes looked misshapen, and her speech was indistinct. I asked her if she knew where she was, and she did. I asked her whether she understood the implications of her transfer, and she nodded. She picked up on my uneasiness and reassured me with a smile that she was pleased to be exactly where she was.

She was peaceful. I was not. The staff nurse said there was

no sign of imminent death and that I should not be worried. She said I should go home and sleep. At 8 p.m., I realised that I hadn't eaten. I walked to a nearby restaurant and ordered pizza and a glass of wine. It made sense to go home, knowing she was comfortable. But something didn't feel right about that. I returned to the hospice.

In the hour I'd been away, her condition had deteriorated. She had fallen into a deep sleep. Her breathing was steady but effortful. Over the next hour, her head fell back, and her mouth remained open as she breathed slowly and loudly. Nurses checked her regularly but said very little. I sat on the two-seater sofa beside her bed and was offered several blankets and pillows. But sleep was out of the question. Around midnight, the nurse confirmed she was dying.

I couldn't do much, but I was happy to be with her and not have her make that journey alone. Letting her be, listening to her making wet crackling sounds, was all she seemed to ask of me.

Many things happened early in my life that fractured the trust between us. We had lots of catching up to do. Sitting by her bed in the hospice, I thought about what still hadn't been said between us. This would be my last chance. I didn't know if she could hear me, but I hoped she could.

I spoke out loud, sometimes through tears. Feelings welled up in me, but I didn't push them away. I felt close to her, which wasn't a feeling I'd often experienced. I accepted her for who she was and her willingness to step bravely into the unknown. She allowed me to open my heart and say what I needed to say.

Keeping my three siblings appraised of Mum's progress wore down my phone battery through the night. As morning broke, I borrowed a charger from the nurses' station and plugged it into the socket at the head of the bed. Later, as I bent down to retrieve it, my face inches from hers, she took her last breath. It was over. She was at peace. And to my surprise, I was too.

We had come full circle. A relationship that had begun and ended with just the two of us, alone and at ease in each other's company. It hadn't ever been easy, but the things that most needed to be said had been said. Her final gift was perhaps the greatest she had ever given me. She showed me how to die. I had watched her for 18 hours walk fearlessly into the night with courage and grace. Never, for a moment, did I get a sense that she looked back. She died well; someday, I hope to honour her by doing the same.

HOME IS WHERE WE START FROM

*Our childhood memories are often fragments, brief
moments or encounters, which together form the
scrapbook of our life. They are all we have left to
understand the story we have come to tell ourselves
about who we are.*[1]

EDITH EGER

Sometimes it's not what we remember that hurts us; it's what we have forgotten. Those painful experiences we've disowned because they were too hard to deal with. We hope that time, even if it doesn't always heal, will eventually give us a safe distance from the past. Whatever hurt us will surely lose its hold on us. Until something happens, and we realise that we haven't outgrown our pain; we've been carrying it with us for years.

I was my parents' first child and the first grandchild in both their families. I was welcomed and loved. My father was in the army, stationed at the time in Cork. My mother was a telephonist until they married. In 1950s Ireland, marriage for a woman meant giving up one's career to stay home and look after the children.

I was born on St Patrick's Hill. We lived in my mother's childhood home in Cork City until my father was reassigned to Dublin nine months later. The army provided him with a three-bedroom house in Villa Park Gardens off the Navan Road. Within a year my brother Jim had arrived, a curly-haired blonde boy with big blue eyes. By all accounts, the four of us were happy in that little house. But in my second year, everything changed.

Jim contracted measles when he was only 16 months old. Measles is a highly contagious infectious viral disease. A tiny percentage of children who develop measles suffer complications, which may be lethal. Jim was one of those unlucky ones. He developed meningitis with secondary encephalitis. He was admitted to Temple Street Children's Hospital early on Sunday morning, 16 May 1955, and died that evening at 10 p.m.

This happened in the 1950s when people didn't talk about the death of a child. In later years, my mother would describe how Jim's death made her a marked woman among young parents on our street. 'They kept their distance,' she said, 'as though whatever I had done to cause Jim to die might be contagious.'

My mother told me much later in my life that she and Dad never talked to each other about their loss. Love, for each of them, meant not hurting the other. They each kept their grief to themselves, believing that to give sorrow words would only have added to the other's distress. When my stoical father returned late from Temple Street Hospital that Sunday night, he said, 'He died, but it was for the best. If he'd lived, he'd have been a vegetable.' They barely referred to Jim again until 1985.

The following day my father left our home alone and asked our next-door neighbour Sean Diffley – the only car owner on our street – to drive him to Temple Street to collect Jim's remains. They parked outside the hospital entrance. Sean waited in the car as my father went in to look for his son. He found a tiny white coffin with the name 'James Bates' hand-written on the lid, beside 16 May 1955. Without even a brief prayer, a religious sister accompanied him as he carried the tiny casket out the front entrance and placed it on the car's back seat.

Neither he nor Sean had any plan for what to do next. They agreed that the only cemetery they were both familiar with was Mount Jerome, near Harold's Cross Bridge, and headed there. When they arrived, they found the place deserted. Without anyone to advise them on what they should do or how they might go about burying a child, they left the coffin under a tree and drove away.

The day Jim died I was a month off my third birthday. I can't remember what I felt about his sudden absence. I've always felt that his death took something from all our lives. Without permission to speak about him in the family, we could not mourn or grieve his loss. The emptiness of his absence seemed to hang in the air as our collective grief became frozen in time. And then, five days after Jim died, I came close to joining him.

My father returned to work after leaving his coffin at Mount Jerome cemetery. For the remainder of that week, he was confined to barracks. The army didn't do compassionate leave in those years. He'd buried his son on Monday and reported for duty that same afternoon.

Finding herself alone with me in an empty house, shattered by the loss of Jim, my mother decided to travel to her family home in Cork. She needed help with looking after me. A few days after we arrived, I came down with rubella and was admitted to the Cork Fever Hospital.

Within 24 hours, I developed secondary encephalitis, just like Jim, and was considered terminal. The doctor meant well when he said to my mother, 'You've already lost one son this week; you don't need to go through the agony of seeing your only other child die. Why don't you go back to Dublin? You can check how he's doing if you can get to a phone. Otherwise, be sure to pick up a daily newspaper. When Tony dies, we'll publish the details in the *Cork Examiner*.'

My mother was a compliant woman. She listened to this doctor and did precisely what he had advised. In her mid-twenties, completely alone, she boarded a train for Dublin. She had lost one child and was about to lose another. That train journey was one of the lowest moments of her life.

Both my parents travelled to Cork to see me the following

weekend. To everyone's surprise, I'd beaten the medic's four-day prognosis. When they came to see me on the ward, I was in a small cot with tall glass on every side. Physical contact was prohibited. I was barely moving in my bed and did not appear interested in communicating with them.

But appearances can be deceptive. When they left the ward, I was inconsolable. So much so that the next day, the staff nurse strongly suggested to my parents that it would be easier on me if they stayed away altogether. There were no more visits until I was discharged four weeks later.

My mother came to take me home on 21 June, my third birthday. Again, I seemed indifferent to her presence. I pushed her away when she tried to hug me. She was hurt that I wasn't happy to see her.

But whatever we lacked in terms of an emotional connection, I was utterly dependent on her physically. I'd regressed in terms of toilet training and speech. My calf muscles had deteriorated. Both my feet and ankles had developed secondary deformities due to my infection. I had to be carried everywhere. I was given to aggressive outbursts and found it impossible to calm myself down.

This was more than my mother could bear. She was a bereaved, depressed, isolated woman with very low self-confidence. The neighbours kept their distance. Her army husband coped with whatever grief he felt by saying nothing. She was pregnant again. It was all too much. She decided I'd be a lot happier back with her family in Cork. I'd always been a hit with her younger siblings; maybe I might open up to them.

She took me to Cork and left me with her parents and siblings for the next six months. I cannot remember how I felt being separated from my mother for such a long time, but I suspect it left me with a feeling of not being wanted – a feeling which was to become a steady companion to me for most of my life. I never talked about my feelings to anyone as a child – probably because no one ever asked – but my behaviour at times suggested that behind my placid mask lived an angry little boy.

In the years following my discharge from the fever hospital, I developed what I can now see were odd behaviours. Around age five, back in Dublin, I took to getting up in the middle of the night and leaving the house without making a sound. I went on a walkabout in the local neighbourhood before dawn, only returning home when the rattle of crates and bottles announced the milkman making his deliveries.

My first school was St. John Bosco's on the Navan Road, which in the late 1950s was a temporary building behind the church. I dreaded having to go there. It was about a half mile from our house in Villa Park Gardens, and I could walk the distance myself. Those were safer times.

My terror was worse on some days than others. When it was particularly bad, I would stand still on the side of the Navan Road across from the school. Usually, I would cross over and pass through the big church gates to get to the school, but on those bad days, I would turn around and make as if to go back home. Of course, I couldn't go home, so I settled on hiding in the warren of lanes that snaked behind the houses lining the main road. Fearful of some adult confronting me, I hid in the shadows and kept out of sight. I remember getting soaked in the rain and taking shelter under trees. As the day progressed, I wandered for about a mile through the building sites and open fields that bordered our neighbourhood.

What made these adventures preferable to being at school is hard to understand. The days were long and unpleasant. My school lunch was my only comfort, and I would typically have it eaten by 10 a.m. In the early days of my mitching, I had no way to get anything else to eat. That changed when I stole some loose change from home to buy sweets from a shop where I wasn't known.

One day stands out for me still. I can see myself walking home at the correct time, having had an accident. I remember vividly turning onto our cul de sac in my short pants, excrement flowing down both legs. I was filled with shame when I arrived home. The litany of lies I told my mother only made me feel worse. When I asked her in later years, she said she had no idea I'd ever missed school.

I look back at photos of myself as a child and see a happy-looking boy. This is confusing as my memories of those years are mostly unhappy. I had too many secrets, and with each year of my childhood, they grew in number.

My feelings for my mother were all mixed up. I knew in

some part of my child's brain that I was holding back from her. Maybe I was furious with her for all the times she'd left me and wanted her to feel the pain that I was feeling. But I couldn't admit my anger; that was much too frightening. I wanted her to smash down the walls between us and comfort me. Probably fearing that my 'bad' feelings would hurt her somehow, I always tried to be a 'good boy' and help her as much as possible. I tidied up after meals, tried to keep my younger siblings in line and emptied ashtrays. I listened as she made the rounds of our bedrooms at night to say good night, longing for her to tuck me in and kiss me. But instead of allowing that to happen, I would turn away from the door, pull the blankets around me and pretend to be asleep. She would open the door, assume I was already asleep, softly close the door and leave.

Living with confusion and turmoil is exhausting and I needed ways to shut down those feelings. Lying, stealing and mitching school didn't make me feel good about myself, but they relieved me momentarily. I built walls to hide 'despicable me' from the world. But I often woke in the middle of the night and felt terrified by something I couldn't put my finger on. Lying awake in the dark, I would listen to distant fog horns. I imagined that sound was made by a little boy, lost at sea and utterly alone in the dark. It never struck me for a moment that the lost boy was myself.

Daydreaming became another refuge from inner chaos. I created worlds full of dangers and threats, which I overcame with exceptional bravery and talent. When I entered primary school, my stories began to centre on some distressed maiden. By age seven or eight, the gallant-knight-rescues-beautiful-young-girl motif had become my favourite bedtime story.

Eilis, a dark-haired girl in my first year of primary school, stole my heart. She needed lots of rescuing, as, unfortunately for her, she was beset nightly by bullies in the lane beside our house as I tried to lull myself to sleep. Naturally, I always recognised her cry for help. I leapt through my bedroom window onto our flat-roofed kitchen; from there, I jumped into the lane alongside our house and imposed myself between her and her predators. My presence alone made them think twice about continuing to threaten her. She never recognised me as the boy from her class, but I hoped that someday we would become best friends.

That same fairy tale had many iterations throughout my life, with different faces stepping in to play the leading lady. Its ability to soothe and comfort could always be counted on.

Learning to read extended the landscape of my imagination. The lady in our local library introduced me to endless characters and adventures. Enid Blyton gave me friends with whom I could spend time. I relished their company and revelled in their adventures. In my mind, they were real people.

Richmal Crompton wrote 39 books in her 'Just William' series, and I read every one. William made me laugh out loud. I lived his every adventure. I marvelled at his total disregard for social convention. He risked social disapproval, which I tried so hard to avoid. He refused to be ashamed when his exploits were exposed as reckless, whereas I knew I would collapse in shame if that happened to me. William was precisely the role model I needed.

Fantasy was a big part of my life. I constantly made up stories where I overcame impossible challenges that earned me admiration and a sense of belonging. I was reassured to read later in my life that children in concentration camps survived by escaping into idealised worlds of their creation:

> When the real world is terrifying, daydreams can give rise to wild hopes that make it bearable. When pain is too great, we can't perceive anything else. We are just in pain. But as soon as we get some distance from it, though stepping into daydreams, imagining a place where everything that has been taken from us or denied is available in abundance. Once we have some distance from our pain, we can transform it into a story or a play. As soon as we can turn our experience into a play or story that makes them bearable.[2]

If the world became too hard to handle, I simply invented another one and spent time there. My imagination became a place where I could plot, plan, and re-invent myself as gifted, powerful, and lovable. The problem with fantasy, however, is that when we rely on it too much, we can become less and less able to deal with reality. We can also lose touch with ourselves. I remember being confused about what was real and what I had made up about myself. As the gap between my ideal and my real self widened, I grew increasingly unable to cope with social situations. I dreaded anyone looking at me and seeing how messed up I was. I imagined if they found out, they would be appalled or, even worse, disappointed.

My childhood wasn't all bad. There were also moments when the company of friends and our various adventures made life not only bearable but wonderful. But most of the time, I hurt inside. My efforts at 'self-soothing' and 'pain management' evolved. I engaged in stranger and more self-destructive behaviours, such as stripping down to my underpants at night and circling my bedroom frantically whilst compulsively biting my knees and elbows. This ritual had ceased by the time I was 10 years old, but for a couple of years, it happened on a regular basis. No one seemed to have any idea what I was doing. Except on one occasion, when I came close to being exposed.

When I was eight years old, I was invited by some of our old neighbours on the Navan Road for an overnight stay. Rita and Paddy had no children, but they'd always been fond of me. Their home seemed plush compared to ours. They had carpets and heavy curtains and delicate-looking ornaments on shelves. I was treated like a prince, and when it was time for bed, I was shown to a very spacious bedroom. We said our good nights and they closed the door. I heard them go back downstairs and, in the distance, I could still hear the TV. Theirs was the first house in my childhood to have a television.

I started to experience feelings I wished I didn't have. My stomach felt hollow; my body was tense. I felt lost, and I didn't know what to do. But then I remembered that 'thing' I would sometimes do. I stripped off my clothes, ran wildly around the bed and when I completed each circuit, I bit and sucked my arms, knees and elbows in a particular order. I did this for nearly an hour, increasing my pace around the bed and biting harder as I worked myself into a compulsive frenzy.

I can see now that finding myself alone in unfamiliar surroundings triggered familiar feelings and sensations that I'd never been able to manage. I made no conscious connection with my past, but my body relived it. Climbing into that large adult bed and turning off the light risked allowing these painful feelings to surface and overwhelm me. This mindless compulsive ritual peppered with self-harm was a preferable alternative. It put distance between me and my distress. Perhaps it was also a way to vent my anger and confusion at finding myself, yet again, far from home and trapped.

Many years later, I discovered that the technical term for how we behave when traumatic sensations are triggered is 'dissociation'. This is one of the ways nature has equipped humans to deal with fear.

The dissociative response is used when there is inescapable, unavoidable distress and pain. Your mind and body protect you. Because you cannot physically flee, and fighting is futile, you psychologically flee to your inner world … a whole set of neurophysiological changes helps you do that, including releasing your body's own opiates.[3]

My frenzy finally exhausted me. I bit myself until I was bruised and bloody, releasing endorphins that soothed me, until I eventually gave up and fell asleep. What I hadn't realised was that my performance had an audience. When I arrived down to breakfast the following day, Paddy and Rita looked at me. Rita enquired tentatively, 'Did you find it hard to get to sleep, love?'

I realised with a feeling of embarrassment that my bedroom was directly above the TV room. They'd had to endure my feet pounding the ceiling for however long it took me to wear myself out. I imagined them looking at each other, unused to the quiet of their nightly TV time being broken in such an unsettling manner.

I don't remember whether I managed to eat breakfast or not. All I know is that I never stayed in their house again.

Another incident that comes to mind occurred the summer I turned nine. As the school year ended, my mother brought me to my grandparent's home, what we called 'the big house' in Cork, intending to leave me there until the end of July. I was put in my grandmother's bedroom the night we arrived. It had a big double bed. There was a box of matches on the bedside table. I took a match from the box, lit it and tossed the lighted match on the bed covers. I did this repeatedly until the sheets caught fire. I felt some strange catharsis as I watched flames rise all around me. They rose higher and higher until they began to lick the wallpaper behind me.

My mother burst into the room. She started screaming. I heard other voices. She grabbed me from the bed and carried me to safety. People rushed in to douse the flames.

That was the first time I saw my mother angry. She was furious. When a crisis had been averted, and control had been restored, she took me to another room in the house, pulled down my pants and gave me a beating. I didn't mind the pain; at that moment, I was getting the best attention I'd had in years. And I loved the assertive, furious, passionate woman she had become. Gone was the overly-apologetic 'nice' lady she'd been in social situations. My self-effacing mother had suddenly become real. Sadly, we soon returned to hiding our pain behind smiles and good manners. Back home in Dublin, she never complained, always looked out for our family, and despite 40 cigarettes a day, enjoyed good physical health. But I was aware of another side of her personality. I noticed how she kept apologising for herself. I heard her crying in her room. I always felt responsible in some way for her distress. I pretended not to notice, but I would try harder to be helpful. I would wash dishes, tidy up, and on one occasion I took out a tin of white paint and painted over stains on the kitchen wall. In our family, it was all about covering over the cracks and keeping up appearances.

In my adolescence, I progressed from stealing loose change from my parents to becoming a small-time thief. It turned out I had a natural flair for shoplifting. Chocolate bars, toffee sweets and biros were among my spoils. I would share them with my classmates to win their friendship. Whoever said 'money can't buy you love' had never met the boys in my school.

My 'funny feet' – secondary deformities from rubella – followed me through primary school into secondary school. From wearing steel braces locked into my shoes until I was four years old, I graduated to 'special' orthopaedic shoes, which I wore until I was fourteen. I attended the Dublin Orthopaedic Hospital throughout my childhood. I crossed the city by bus three times weekly, alone, from age eight. That hospital was on Merrion Square in the building that is now the Merrion Hotel. The clinic I attended was a prefabricated building at the end of the back garden. I still remember the smell of feet as I opened the door. My sessions involved a routine of painful exercises. Afterwards, I caught the number 20 bus home from Stephen's Green. Sitting upstairs in smoke-filled buses on dark evenings, I used my sleeve to clear fogged-up windows so I could see where we were and not miss my stop.

This regime did nothing for my reputation at school. I couldn't participate in mandatory sports activities and was the target of serious schoolboy resentment when I left school early, three days every week, to attend rehab. I think I was tolerated because I was a reliable source of chocolate and biros.

Pornography was added to the list of hidden behaviours that formed my secret life. Forbidden copies of *Parade* and *Playboy* passed around by friends were soothing, addictive and also deeply troubling – something else to tighten the grip of shame. A more open, candid sex education programme might have helped, but pornography seemed to meet a need that I didn't understand and that I doubt anybody else could have understood at the time. It simulated intimacy of a kind of which I was starved.

In my later years of primary school, there were occasions when my mother and I would be home alone. Sometimes she would look at me with a strained expression and tell me how bitterly she regretted some things that happened when I was little. She never said what they were, but she feared those memories would return to me someday, and I would hate her. I had no idea what she was talking about.

Until one day, many years later, when something triggered my body's memories and brought me face to face with a 'me' I didn't know and didn't want to know.

2

IN SEARCH OF SELF

It's hard to remember adolescence. The worry, havoc, and pure joy of breaking out into the world.[1]

ANNIE ROGERS

My adolescence began with a mysterious illness. There was probably an underlying medical reason for my condition, but our family GP, Paddy Smith, was always puzzled by my symptoms. The explanation that he finally agreed upon with my parents was that it had been triggered by a severe chill I'd experienced a few weeks before.

On a windy Saturday afternoon in January of my first year of secondary school, I was cycling along the Clontarf seafront when I noticed a group of adults staring out over the low sea wall. I parked and joined them out of curiosity. I was struck by how high the tide was on the far side of the waterfront. White spray stung my eyes as the wind churned up waves and splashed water onto the path where we stood.

As I adjusted my slit eyes to the squalls, I understood what had stopped this little community on their afternoon stroll. Their gaze was fixed on an object bobbing up and down in the frenzied water. It wasn't a person, as I instinctively assumed it must be. It was a large grey and white Alsatian dog, a particular breed I immediately recognised as I had always been terrified of them. It was struggling to stay afloat 20 to 30 feet beyond our reach.

Somebody should do something, I thought. Despite his best efforts at swimming, the dog was being carried further out to sea. The innocent animal was going to drown. *Somebody should do something.*

I was a less-than-mediocre swimmer but had completed some school-sponsored life-saving classes in Tara Street Baths. Without much deliberation, I took off the precious army coat – dyed brown and fitted with bronze buttons – that had passed down from my grandfather. It functioned as both an identity statement and a security blanket. Entrusting my coat, scarf and shoes to some anonymous bystander, I lowered myself down a rusty steel ladder fixed to the outer wall, holding a life ring under one of my arms.

The cold was numbing. I fought against fierce waves that seemed intent on keeping me pinned to the wall. I swam in the direction of the dog with immense effort. My progress was slow, and the dog's distress was rising. I sensed it was exhausted when I reached it and needed some buoyancy assistance. If I could secure the life ring around its body, I knew it had a rope held at the other end by someone on shore.

The dog was having none of it. It didn't seem the least

happy to see me. He or she fought me every step of the way as I tried to guide it to shore. I don't know how we made it. I remember the crowd hauling the sodden dog out of the water up and over the wall and hands reaching down to pull me out also.

People said nice things to me, but everyone left after a very short time. One man promised to alert the Gardaí to what had happened and to tell them where they could find the dog and me. We both sat on the green beside the footpath and waited. The rain had stopped. It was getting dark. We were both shivering, the dog looking worse than I did. So, I wrapped my coat around its drenched body.

By five o'clock, I had started to worry. Then I saw a Garda motorcycle driving towards us. He pulled up beside us and took down my details. We were within a mile of the nearest Garda station, and he assured me that either a car or van would come and take us there within the hour. All seemed right with the world. Sometimes the good guys do show up to save the day.

We waited. The sky grew dark, and the wind cut through me. I wanted to retrieve my coat but was more concerned with the dog's welfare than my own. I heard the Angelus bell ring in the local Catholic church. It was six o'clock, and I was expected home for dinner.

We continued to wait. Nobody came, despite my telling myself they would. After sitting there for another hour, I finally admitted that help wasn't coming for either of us.

I started walking towards the Garda station through the dark. When we arrived, I recognised the interior décor as I'd been there once before, after breaking a neighbour's front window with a rock. At the time I had tried to plead my innocence, saying it had been a long front garden, and I seriously did not believe I could throw a rock of that size that far (even though I had put my best into taking that shot and felt some pride in my achievement). The Garda looking at the soaking, shivering pair standing in his reception that day didn't seem any more friendly than the one who greeted me on my previous visit.

He took the dog and promised to take care of it. I headed straight home, conscious that I was late for dinner. I looked a mess, so I snuck upstairs to my bedroom to change before I joined the family. Dad was minding us that weekend as Mum was in hospital. I feared he would not be impressed if I told the truth about my exploits that afternoon; the last thing he wanted was for me to get into trouble on his watch. So I acted as though nothing had happened.

Whenever my mother was absent, Dad always resorted to Beshoff's for takeaway fish and chips. The original shop was established by Anthony Beshoff, a few doors down from our home on Malahide Road.

That particular Sunday, there were more leftovers than usual. I asked if I could share them with a 'friend'. My request provoked a series of questions, and the story of my hair-brained rescue trickled out. My father hardly reacted at all.

It was impossible to know whether he was cross with me for being irresponsible or impressed with me for trying to do the right thing.

I bagged my booty and carried it enthusiastically to the Garda station. There was a different Garda at reception. He didn't seem any more pleased to see me than the last guy. I recounted my rescue story, to which he replied, 'Oh, that dog was taken away and put down early this morning.'

My heroics were for nothing. My only reward was a mysterious illness two weeks later that grounded me for over half that school year. Looking back, I'm not convinced that my ailments were entirely physical. But our GP decided I had, or was seriously at risk of, rheumatic fever. He respected my mother's opinion and agreed to a six-month course of penicillin and bed rest.

I must have experienced a sense of déjà vu during those months. Once again, I was alone in a bed, semi-immobilised and separated from my everyday life. Was my body trying to re-live an old story and give it a better outcome this time? Or was my extended bed rest more to do with my mother? Maybe she wanted me in a place where she could care for me, as I usually made that impossible. Bedrest was her go-to remedy for every ailment. And, once again, I was physically unable to perform basic functions independently. She had to carry me in and out of the bathroom for the first few weeks of my recuperation. That can't have been easy for a 13-year-old boy, but I have no memory of resisting her help.

I didn't miss school, although I remember feeling vaguely guilty as I listened to normal life building slowly to a frenetic pace outside my window every morning. My physical world shrank to the dimensions of my box room, but an inner landscape opened with limitless frontiers. Books mapped new adventures. I became immersed in works like *Treasure Island* and *Kidnapped*, not knowing at the time that they were written by someone who had also endured years in bed as a child.

When I resumed school the following September, I was dropped from the A to the B stream. Because I had a talent for maths and English, I was told to attend the A-stream classes in those specific subjects, where I could continue to study them at honours level. My daily shifting between the A and B streams for the remainder of my secondary education was like a bad metaphor for my life. I didn't belong anywhere.

That summer I stepped out of my bed into the mid-1960s. Into a time when our collective human consciousness was stretched beyond the cosy confines of accepted convention. Martin Luther King insisted on equality in the face of the vile racism that had become normal practice across the United States. War, condoned by a majority during the 1940s, was challenged in the wake of our growing realisation that the scars of the battlefield remain long after the shooting stops. The Beatles, Pink Floyd and the Beach Boys re-defined rock music. In Rome, the pope convened Vatican II and rewrote the rules for engaging with God. No paradigm, creed or cultural practice went unchallenged. The Apollo moon landing symbolised a generation's desire to go beyond limits felt to have been imposed on it for too long.

As teenagers, being different – even outrageous – was the new normal. The sober attire of the past was traded in for paisley shirts, bellbottoms and miniskirts. Our emerging identities were colourful and expansive. We despised our parents 'better-to-be-safe-than-sorry' wisdom and opted instead for risk and innovation. We listened to cultural icons who prided themselves on their use of drugs, guilt-free sex and high-risk behaviours. If we could travel to the dark side of the moon, we should not be afraid of darker elements in ourselves. All we needed was love, and it was everywhere.

The 1960s can be faulted for its excesses, but what redeemed it was the way it constantly appealed to the natural idealism latent in young people. Success was still important, but the new attitude was that it should be measured in creative rather than merely economic terms, by what we contributed to society rather than just what we achieved for ourselves.

My adolescence was full of experimentation and idealism. By the time I entered university, I had become immersed in a vibrant world of music, romance, spirituality and social change. The gap between my experimental self and the boy in me who continued to feel lost widened. Allowing the gap between our private and public selves to grow can impact our mental health. We may survive for long periods by living in different worlds, acting quite differently in each. But eventually, a time comes when the gap between our contradictory selves becomes too hard to maintain, and we fall apart.

I searched song lyrics and soulful writings for words and insights I could relate to. Paul Simon and Jim Morrison made me feel I was not weird. The truths they captured became handrails I grasped to get me through life. Music touched me in ways I had never been touched before. I also found consolation in the works of Hesse, Mann, Bellow and Solzhenitsyn, which gradually replaced the likes of Robert Louis Stephenson, Daniel Defoe and Arthur Conan Doyle by my bedside.

My father was a gregarious man. He loved meeting people but found it hard to relax around them. My younger brother, Mel, once described him as a man who used talk to defeat conversation. He could feel very awkward in social situations. He talked endlessly to cover his shyness and had opinions on every subject. People liked him a lot. He was always good company. But he seemed incapable of discussing anything of an emotional nature.

When I finished secondary school, he told me that, in his view, there were basically three choices when it came to a university education: medicine, engineering and arts. 'An arts degree,' he said dismissively, 'isn't worth much.' Apparently, it restricted rather than expanded one's career options later in life. That left two alternatives. I wasn't talented with my hands, which eliminated engineering as an option. And I had spent several years in The Order of Malta and enjoyed caring for people injured on football pitches, at carnivals or during large social events. So, I chose medicine.

I lived a colourfully adventurous life on the outside, but my inner world became more insecure with every passing year. My intensity short-circuited any relationship with romantic potential, as the latest object of my affection soon figured out that something was a little 'off' about me. Who wants to be with someone who is always talking big ideas and yet seems so damn nervous when it comes to the business of intimacy?

My thinking then was convoluted and splintered. My lack of coherence was evident in my journals. Here is a typical entry I made when I was about to turn 19. If coherence is a marker of our mental health, then I wasn't in a great place when I wrote this:

So much insecurity and confusion. About everything. I sit here smoking, not knowing what the right thing would be for me to do today and not feeling very much anyway. I keep asking myself about my personality. What is it? Does it reflect what I am? If the latter, then maybe it's right to be weak and confused with others. At least that would seem honest … I wonder if my need for people – my need to meet and talk to them – is a way of escaping from working things out on my own. If that's so, I must close the doors for a while.

Failing to make it at home, in college and in my relationships, I turned to God to save me. Nothing else had managed to give me a sustainable identity. I joined prayer meetings, made a retreat in Taizé and earnestly prayed that I had a vocation. If I couldn't make it as a human being in the real world, maybe I could survive as a monk.

Spirituality allowed me to experience moments where I was more than just 'me'. Moments of internal liberation when I escaped my inner darkness. So what if I suffered periods of profound embarrassment as I gathered my first-year medicine class to share with them the difference finding Jesus had made in my life? So what if I got my lip split open after approaching a skinhead on O'Connell Bridge in Dublin to tell him how everything he was looking for could be found by simply inviting Jesus into his heart? I was out there, living, doing something with my life. I got to accompany large groups on my guitar pouring their hearts into songs like 'They'll Know We Are Christians By Our Love'.

It's easy to mock the naivety and innocence of simple faith. Many people wrote me off at the time. I experienced occasions where my enthusiasm was mocked, and I was violently disowned by some groups who didn't share my beliefs. It was as if I had woken up one day to find that I could only speak in Chinese, and very few people I spoke to could make sense of what I was saying.

My memories of 'witnessing for Jesus' make me cringe now. I was high, omnipotent, expansive and manic. As that phase of my life followed months of feeling depressed, I would most likely have been classified as bipolar had I been referred to psychiatry at the time. But I prefer to think of those years as an important part of a search for myself. We find ourselves by living our lives, making mistakes and learning from them – not by always playing it safe, being reasonable and keeping our heads down.

Other adults tried to reason with me and propose that if I did need God, I should express my faith within the more socially acceptable practices of the Catholic Church, in which I had been raised. But one person who didn't do this was my father's sister, my aunt Marie Raymond, a Mercy nun in charge of St Lawrence's ward in the Mater Hospital, Dublin.

From my earliest childhood, I had always felt her respect. Whenever my family visited her, she would have a surprise for me – usually a tin of biscuits or a box of chocolates. In my mind, she was obviously a wealthy person to be able to afford such a constant supply of gifts. In those days, treats were much rarer than they are now.

When I found God, I was sure my aunt would be pleased. After all, this was the same God she'd dedicated her life to. Soon after being 'reborn,' I visited the Mater to tell her my good news. She behaved exactly as she always did; she was delighted to see me and arranged tea and biscuits in her office.

She listened intently to all I had to say without interrupting. She asked me about my newfound insights and how I was getting on with the family, my medical studies at UCD and my friends. I vaguely remember being surprised that she didn't want to talk more about God. I had a lot of fresh theological insights to share that might have been useful to her. She listened as I spoke in a much less inhibited way than I normally would. I can still feel her presence, her slight stoop in the chair beside me, her silence as she dropped her gaze to the floor now and then, the softness of her voice when she spoke, the way she replied to what I said evenly without overreacting to anything I said. At some point, I had the fleeting thought that maybe my experience was exceptional. Maybe I had breached accepted theological boundaries and discovered some new landscape of faith that was entirely unknown to her.

Reflecting on that conversation I remember, through tears of gratitude, how beautifully she held me in that moment. While I may have looked and sounded like I was on top of the world, she knew I was in great pain. My mind was reaching beyond its darkness for some light. I was frantically trying to hold my life together. She knew what I was able to hear and what I was simply unable to hear. She knew that being with me, being fully present in a way that only she could be without reacting to or challenging my unsettling revelations, was exactly what I needed. Her presence made me feel that whatever I had to say was far less important than my knowing that I was still loved by her.

My biochemistry professor was less sympathetic a month later at my oral examination. His opening question confused me: 'What would you like to talk about?' I wondered if it was the man's deepest soul speaking to me, and answered, 'Life and what it's all about.' He looked at me crossly and replied, 'I meant carbohydrates, proteins or fats!'

'Ma' Coakley, the anatomy professor, was even more annoyed when she read my response to an exam question concerning the lower arm. I had missed some of her lectures and was singularly ignorant of that specific area of human anatomy. I felt I should apologise and explain why I couldn't answer her question, so I wrote her a personal letter in the answer booklet and added some life-changing theological truths I'd discovered that academic year. I failed both subjects and the entire year.

Feeling unable to face the repeat exams I would have to sit that summer, I decided to drop out of medicine. The following October, in breach of several university rules regarding transferring faculties, I signed up for an arts degree in English, psychology and philosophy. I hoped I might find answers there to my pressing ideological concerns. I had no idea at the time how this decision would shape the rest of my life.

3

TEENAGE DREAMS

My troubled teens coincided with the atrocities we called 'the Troubles' in Northern Ireland. In 1971, the British government introduced internment in response to a significant escalation of violence on the part of the IRA. This involved the mass arrest and imprisonment-without-trial of people suspected of being involved in that organisation.

I was 19 and halfway through the first year of my arts degree at UCD when a request came to our Students for Peace group for two people to travel to Belfast and house-sit for the Vatican Radio correspondent. She had been recalled to Rome for a week and feared leaving an unoccupied house in the middle of a known IRA community. The likelihood was that it would be taken over and used as a safe house for paramilitaries. This request was hard to refuse, coming on the heels of our march on the British Embassy the week before. A Holy Rosary nun, Sr Nora, and I volunteered immediately and caught a train to Belfast the next day.

The journalist's home was a modest semi-detached two-bedroom house on Glenalina Road, Ballymurphy. An open passageway on one side of the house led to a small back garden. Behind that lay the Divis flats, the scene of many clashes with the British Army.

On our first morning there, we woke to gunshots. We ran downstairs and took cover under the dining room table. When the shooting stopped, we re-surfaced and made breakfast. We didn't think much of what had happened, accepting that it was probably routine for the area.

Later that morning, we tidied the house, prepared a fire for that evening when we returned and set off to visit some of our neighbours. The Order of the Missionaries of Charity – Mother Teresa's nuns – had recently moved to Springhill Avenue, only a few streets away. We also wanted to meet Fr Des Wilson, a peace activist pioneering reconciliation between Protestants and Catholics.

When we returned to Glenalina Road, I reached into my jacket pocket for the front door key and discovered that I didn't have it. I'd either lost it or left it behind me. This wasn't the kind of community where you left a spare key under the doormat or even with a friendly neighbour. It was growing dark, and we were both feeling the cold.

I looked up to the front bedroom where I'd spent the night and spotted a potential solution. I hadn't fully closed the small awning window above the main one. If I could climb up and open that window, it was possible that I could reach down on the inside and lift the handle of the main window, which would let me in.

Thankfully, there was a small protruding cover above the front door, which provided a means to access the second-storey window ledge. The only problem was that Saracenarmoured personnel carriers patrolled the streets regularly and we didn't want to attract their attention. We waited in the shadows on the strip of grass running along the side of the house until we saw one pass. After that, the road was completely empty. I decided to take my chances. I climbed onto the cover over the front door and made my way to the window ledge. I stabilised myself before lowering my arm inside the awning window. Just as I felt my right hand grip the inside handle of the main window, I heard a sound I recognised – the roar of a Saracen engine. It was turning into our street and accelerating towards me. What the occupants of that vehicle saw was a man in a green rain jacket 'breaking into' a home on one of the most dangerous streets in Belfast. Their reaction wasn't indifference.

I opened the window, slipped into the bedroom and caught my breath. I tried to slow my heart rate as I walked down the stairs. Seeing the fire I had prepared earlier, I took a moment to find a match and light it up. Then I walked to the front door and opened it.

The first thing I noticed was a soldier lying on the small front lawn with his rifle pointing at the house on the opposite side of the street. Next, I noticed armed soldiers running up the side passage with guns pointed toward the back garden. Finally, I saw the machine gun atop the Saracen pointing right at me.

From my left, I heard a male voice asking, 'Have you just arrived here?' Not an unreasonable question. As he stepped into view, I saw a slim, young soldier with a soft hat. His right arm was outstretched, and he was pointing a pistol at my face. Wanting to be as accurate as possible, I said 'No'. After all, we had arrived the day before. Nora answered at precisely the same time and said 'Yes'. He cocked his pistol. 'Is it yes, or no?' he asked suspiciously. 'And you have southern accents. What's going on here?'

I was petrified. The image that came to my mind at that moment was of Jewish men, women and children walking without protest into the gas chambers of Auschwitz. I had seen black-and-white footage when I was 11 years old and wondered why they were so compliant. Surely they knew what was about to happen? Why didn't they do something? At that moment, I understood their compliance perfectly. I would have done whatever this soldier asked me out of sheer terror. I was petrified. But even more than fear, I felt ashamed of my powerlessness to answer him.

Nora was made of sterner stuff and spoke for both of us. She detailed how, when and why we had arrived and mislaid the key. He lowered his gun. Nora recommended he check if the journalist had told his commander that she'd be out of town that week. Before leaving, he thoroughly searched the place. He remained suspicious.

Later on, we heard a knock at the door. It was the same soldier, but this time he was more friendly. The journalist had indeed left word that her home was being minded by university students from Dublin when she was out of town.

We invited him in, and he stayed a while, grateful for a chance to talk.

He explained that earlier that morning, shots were fired at his squad as they passed our house. It turned out they had come from the Divis flats behind us, but it had seemed too much of a coincidence when they spotted me climbing into the upper-storey window. He was 22 years old, with the rank of Lieutenant, and had eight men under him aged from 18 to 21 years. He hated this assignment. They set out every morning to 'protect' a community that despised them, always knowing one or more of them could be injured or killed. It wasn't why he had joined the army, but he had no choice in where he was assigned. He was genuinely open and friendly, and by the time he left, he was apologising for the fright he'd given us earlier.

The week in Belfast left me feeling rattled. What I learned from it was just how impossible it was to maintain any sense of neutrality or objectivity in such a conflict. Depending on whom you spoke to, you were given a view of the 'other side' as vicious, mean, hateful and violent. Had I been compelled to live in that part of Belfast for any reason, I don't believe I could have survived as a reasonable, neutral peacemaker. At some point, I would have been forced to take sides.

I'm not sure whether it was my experience in Belfast or something else, but two weeks later, I fell apart. This time, I had no way to rationalise my breakdown. I was totally confused and took to the hills – literally. I caught the St Kevin's bus to Glendalough, a national park located in the Wicklow mountains, about 60 kilometres south of Dublin City.

I used the only money I had to pay my fare and realised too late that I had nothing left to pay for food or accommodation. It was early spring, but the weather was cold and wet.

I spent two nights and three days there, walking through the woods, exploring the medieval monastic settlement and sitting by the lake. For shelter, I broke into a boarded-up clubhouse via a roof light just wide enough to slip through. It was empty and dark, but it had a kind of camper bed inside I lay on it fully clothed and wearing my long army coat.

I discovered a discarded whiskey bottle which had about half a shot left in it. I filled it to the top with spring water and rationed it as long as I could. I had no idea what I was doing there and no plan for returning home. I just wandered, my mind full of dismal thoughts about my life. But on the third day, I had an epiphany of sorts as I walked yet another nature trail.

Maybe it was being in such a mystical place, maybe it was the clarity that comes after a long fast. Or maybe it's what happens when we go to some edge in our lives where everything is on the line. But on day three, it hit me: I needed people. That may not sound earth-shattering, but it struck me with the force of a lightning bolt.

I realised that the price I'd paid for hiding under cloaks of shame and behind masks of fear was that I'd become trapped inside my own private hell. Holding firm to some irrational nonsense that I should be able to manage my life without assistance, I had denied my need for relationships. I suffered in isolation and wondered why my life was so hard.

But on that third day in Glendalough, the psychological rock in my mind was rolled back to give me a new clarity about my life. I needed people, I couldn't go it alone. And that was OK.

I felt my energy returning and, with it, a desire to connect more openly with my friends. I made my way to the main road and hitched a ride to Dublin. I was dropped off in the city centre and went directly to the bank, where my friend Carl would soon be taking his lunch break.

After eating lunch – which he graciously treated me to – we stood at the bottom of Grafton Street outside his bank. He asked me what I wanted to do next. I pointed to the Irish Permanent Building Society offices on the corner of Grafton and Nassau Street and said, 'I want to buy that building and turn it into a place where young people like me can turn when they need to talk to someone.'

There are moments in our lives when we have a vision of something we would love to do because it makes so much sense to us, and we feel we have what it takes to make it happen. It may seem that my idea then was nothing more than a teenage dream, but it came in a moment of absolute clarity. I was 19, experiencing some form of breakdown, and had no qualifications or resources. But I saw what needed to be done to support young people like me. It would take another 30 years, but I would eventually make that idea a reality.

Teenage dreams are hard to beat.

4

LEARNING TO LISTEN

*The purest form of listening is to listen without
memory or desire.*[1]

WILFRED BION

As part of my second-year psychology degree course,
we were asked to watch a short black-and-white film
on a concept known as 'attachment theory', called 'A
Two-Year-Old Goes to Hospital'. This proved to be a critical
personal and professional milestone in my life.

Attachment theory emerged in the 1950s and was based
largely on the work of John Bowlby, a British psychoanalyst.[2]
It shifted the focus of psychology from the dynamics of the
unconscious to the fundamental importance of how we were
cared for in our early childhood. Bowlby observed aspects
of the mother–child relationship that give human beings the
essential security to live their lives. Healthy attachment –
based on attentive and responsive parenting – enables a child
to trust themselves (autonomy) and form deep and lasting
relationships with others (intimacy). Failure to experience
security in infancy leaves us with problems achieving both.

Attachment theory speaks to something fundamental to all of us. We all need love and are hard-wired to seek it throughout our lives. We need to feel close, to be held, to feel needed. A secure relationship with others is how we ground our lives and find the energy and passion for living.

James Robertson, who worked with Bowlby, made the film I watched 20 years later in UCD.[3] Robertson was a registered conscientious objector in the Second World War. In 1941, he and his partner, Joyce, joined Anna Freud in the Hampstead War Nursery to help Anna look after war orphans. Joyce was a student nurse who cared directly for the infants, and James was responsible for building maintenance and fire watch.

Anna Freud's policy was that every worker in the hospital, regardless of their title or role, shared responsibility for the children under their care. She required everyone to notice any child with whom they interacted and submit their observations to her in writing at the end of the day. Robertson complied and became so interested in the work that he enrolled for a degree in social work after the war. He graduated in 1948 as a psychiatric social worker. He was particularly concerned for children who became separated from their parents. A year later, he joined John Bowlby at the Tavistock clinic to further his studies.

As part of his post-graduate training, Robertson was assigned to a short-stay children's ward at the Central Middlesex Hospital in London. He was shocked by the unhappiness he saw among these children, particularly those under the age of three. The staff executed their duties competently but seemed unaware of the distress around them. They believed that while children were initially upset at being separated from their parents, they seemed to settle fine after a few days and do whatever they were told to do. Robertson interpreted their behaviour in a very different way.

He observed three distinct phases in a child's reaction to separation: protest, despair and denial/detachment. In the protest phase, the child is visibly distressed, gets angry, cries and calls for their mother. If the child is reunited with their mother at this stage, they will usually be quite ambivalent towards her, as though they want to punish the mother for going away.

If the separation continues for longer, the child's distress turns to despair. They become reticent, withdrawn, miserable and apathetic. They lose interest in everything. They may appear to be 'settling down' to the satisfaction of an unenlightened staff. But for Robertson, this emotional withdrawal reflected an effort to shut down the pain of potentially never seeing their mother again.

In the denial/detachment phase, the child shows more interest in his surroundings, interacts with others, and if reunited at this stage, will seem indifferent towards their mother coming or going. This is why Robertson regarded detachment as the most detrimental phase. It was as though the child managed to survive the separation by 'killing off their love for the mother.'[4]

Robertson's observations were met with hostility by the medical profession. Even his colleagues at the Tavistock clinic did not share his belief that enforced separation, with severely restricted visits, was distressing for children under three. They misinterpreted the compliance of the quiet, withdrawn child as evidence of their adjustment to separation. They couldn't see what he saw.

Robertson came up with an idea to open their eyes. He would film what was happening on the ward. With a grant of £150, he purchased a cine camera and 80 minutes of black-and-white film. He had never used a cine camera before. The resulting film, 'A Two-Year-Old Goes to Hospital', has been designated of national and historical importance. A copy is preserved in the National Archives of the United Kingdom.

In the film, Laura, aged two, is hospitalised for eight days for a minor operation. She is too young to understand her mother's absence. Because her mother is not there and the nurses change frequently, she has to face the fears, frights and hurts of a medical procedure and a new environment with no familiar person to cling to. She is distraught by a rectal anaesthetic. After a time, she becomes quiet and 'settles'. On discharge, she is withdrawn and indifferent to her mother.

As I watched the film, a burning panic spread throughout my body. I found breathing hard and had to get out of the lecture hall. Watching it shook me, but I had no idea why. At the time, I could only remember being in the hospital on two occasions when I was five and eight years old. They were brief admissions – both to the Mater Hospital. My Aunty Raymond, was in charge of St Laurence's ward and had made sure I was well-minded. While I remembered not being happy there, I didn't think it was traumatic.

I had repressed any memory of my time in Cork Fever Hospital when I was two. That file was sealed and hidden deep in the recesses of my unconscious. But while the mind can keep things hidden, even from ourselves, the body never forgets. I resonated viscerally with Laura's sadness in the film. Watching her slip into despair, I experienced a spasm of pain as vividly as if it had been me in that cot instead of her, but I had no idea why.

Studying psychology suited me. Early in my life, I discovered that what was hidden inside us, usually something painful, often something shameful, lay at the root of most of our suffering. I knew what this could do to a person. I was ripe for a career that helped others do what I was desperately trying to do for myself: gather up the broken pieces of my life and make sense of inner chaos.

If the human spirit hovers somewhere between earth and heaven, psychology chooses to stay close to the ground. It asks fundamental questions about behaviour. How do we learn? How do we form ideas and develop our intelligence? How do we cope with the sorrows and setbacks we encounter? What happens when the mind loses touch with reality? How do relationships work, and why do they often not?

I stepped into psychology with a bachelor's degree at age 23. I knew very little. I was offered a trainee psychologist position at Cluain Mhuire Family Centre in Blackrock. This included permission to complete a master's degree in applied psychology at UCD. I spent two days a week working with children and a day each week working with the adolescent and adult teams, respectively. I attended my college courses on Fridays.

In that same year, Ursula and I married. I had met Ursula at the beginning of our third year in college. We got to talking in a very animated way at our first meeting and were surprised to discover we were on the same psychology course. Our relationship moved from a deep friendship at the beginning of the year to something much deeper by the end of that academic year. We were engaged within six months and married the following summer. She signed up for a full-time master's degree while I started in Cluain Mhuire. We started our life together in a one-room flat on Newtownpark Avenue, opposite where I worked. Then, in 1978, we had our first child Andrew and moved to our first home in Marsham Court, Stillorgan.

In the late 1970s, the role of a psychologist was narrowly defined. We were perceived as technicians who administered psychological tests. These instruments allowed us to measure a person's level of intelligence, memory, how well their brain was functioning and their coping styles.

David Weschler, who developed the most popular IQ

test, played an important role in gaining credibility for psychologists. Wechsler was a Romanian Jew who migrated to the USA as a child and graduated as a psychologist in 1917, at the peak of America's involvement in the First World War. In 1932, he was made chief psychologist at Bellevue Psychiatric Hospital in New York, where he stayed for 35 years.[5]

Wechsler was concerned for Bellevue's patients and wanted to capture their unique strengths and weaknesses. At that time, psychological testing was in its infancy. All that was available was the Binet Scale. This was a test which offered a single measure of a person's level of intelligence, referred to as their intelligence quotient or IQ. Wechsler didn't like this test because it didn't allow for the scope of human intelligence. He thought of intelligence not as something we *have* but as something we *do*, our capacity 'to act purposefully, to think rationally and to deal effectively with the environment'.

He developed the Weschler Adult Intelligence Scale (WAIS) as an alternative to the Binet Scale. This new measure consisted of 11 short tests assessing verbal and non-verbal intelligence. Wechsler hoped that the results achieved on his tests would reveal a unique personal profile of strengths and limits. In a world where psychiatric patients were written off as uniformly 'mad', this was his attempt to profile the uniqueness of each individual, regardless of their diagnosis.

I liked Weschler's scale because it allowed the tester to see how a person tackled problems. While administering the children's version of his intelligence test, I soon discovered that a child's test behaviour was far more important than their numerical scores. For example, some children loved the verbal 'question-and-answer' subtests, which allowed them to interact with me. However, the same child might flounder in response to the non-verbal subtests, where they were assigned a task and left silently to their own devices. The inevitable discrepancy between their verbal and non-verbal scores spoke less of a lack of intelligence, pointing instead towards emotional issues that made autonomy difficult or threatening. The opposite presentation was equally common. A child would avoid eye contact and give only minimal responses to verbal tests but become immersed in non-verbal tasks and score significantly higher, raising the possibility that interpersonal trust was an issue for them.

I always met with the parents of these children when we had completed testing. Generally, this meant meeting with their mother, who was usually terrified of having to take her child to see a psychologist. These women spoke candidly about their concerns for their child's welfare and often described a home situation far from ideal. They felt inadequate as parents; the last thing they needed was a professional to add to their guilt. Instinctively, I knew they needed reassurance that they were doing a good enough job as a mother (or, sometimes, a father). I made a habit of opening parent interviews with a remark, such as 'Whatever you're doing with X, he/she is a great kid; they're doing their very best to make a go of life.' Their relief was palpable.

Most children were automatically listed for a repeat assessment six months later. The same parent would often return with that child and say something like, 'Whatever you did with him last time, he's doing so much better. Thank you.' Of course, I had done nothing except treat the parents with respect and remind them they were doing something right. Sometimes the faith we have in each other becomes self-fulfilling.

Overall, though, I felt those assessments achieved very little for the child. Whenever I visited schools and was shown a copy of my report, the final sentence with whatever cumulative 'IQ score' they achieved was highlighted with a yellow marker. Nobody seemed interested in the bigger picture. I imagine the equivalent today would be finding some diagnostic label highlighted, while the unique profile of a child's strengths and struggles that emerged across hours of assessment are ignored.

When it came to adult assessments, personality tests also played a key role. These tests were very different to the Wechsler scales. Projective tests, like the Rorschach Inkblot Test, present a person with something highly ambiguous and invite them to make sense of it. Since the object holds no intrinsic meaning, the only way to give it meaning is for someone to 'project' something from within themselves. Psychologists were divided into those who saw projective tests as useful clinical tools and those who regarded them as lacking any credibility. Following our graduation, Ursula and

I trained with a renowned exponent of the Rorschach test and psychoanalyst Theodora Alcock. Her view of the Rorschach test was that its ambiguity evoked our personal perceptual style and revealed how we made sense of our world and coped with difficult issues. For example, responses dominated by aggressive themes suggested a person's difficulty in handling their rage.

In her classes, Theodora often quoted the Nobel prize-winning neurophysiologist, Charles Sherrington, to explain the basis and importance of the Rorschach test: 'The perceiving mind and the perceived world is all we have. It is the sum total of each of us. They are all we have.'[6]

Psychological testing was an investigative discipline rather than one of technical measurement. There was usually confusion around the people I was asked to assess, and my job was to make sense of their feelings and behaviours and identify issues that needed to be addressed in that person's life. I wrote psychological profiles – stories – that integrated a person's childhood experiences, resulting emotional vulnerabilities, cognitive strengths and shortcomings, and some tentative explanation for the particular distress and behaviour that had led to their admission. I ended with some practical suggestions as to what issues might be usefully explored with them in their recovery.

For the most part, my mini-biographies were not appreciated. The people I wrote them for were more interested in being told a particular patient's diagnosis. Our mental health culture didn't encourage or equip staff to adopt a more personal approach to helping people address unresolved issues.

The rather superficial approach to the complexities of emotional struggles in psychiatry always troubled me. But I lacked the confidence to challenge what others accepted as a professional standard of care. As a rookie psychologist, I was accused of over-complicating things. I was often told that some people were mentally ill, plain and simple, and unlikely to be cured. Our hospital service was there to subdue psychological pain rather than to resolve it. Medication – preferably long-term – would keep a person's emotional life in check.

On my own initiative, I began running groups in St James's for people with common problems. I ran different groups for people with anxiety and low self-esteem, a group on 'healing our inner child' and a practical group that prepared people for discharge. I always co-conducted these groups with someone else, preferably someone who worked in that particular area. My group therapy training was largely from books and the odd professional workshop I attended with visiting practitioners.

My boss, Professor Marcus Webb, encouraged me to sign up for formal psychotherapy training wherever I could find it. He was extraordinarily generous and supportive. He allowed me to research centres of excellence myself and gave me extended leave, with salary, to complete a course of my choice. I travelled to Philadelphia to study formally under

Professor Arron (Tim) Beck, who had developed a new form of psychotherapy known as cognitive behavioural therapy, also known as CBT.

The Center for Cognitive Therapy at the University of Pennsylvania was the centre of the psychotherapeutic field in 1981. Research had shown this new form of therapy to be as effective as antidepressant medications for depression and more protective than drugs against relapse. Beck had also just published his classic tome, *Cognitive Therapy for Depression*, which described how his approach worked in detail.[7] However, when Beck invited me to meet him personally, I knew virtually nothing about the man or his work. All I knew of cognitive therapy was that it was a novel approach that focused more on the present than it did on exploring a person's past.

When I was introduced to Beck, I saw a refined white-haired gentleman wearing a grey linen suit, white shirt and red dickie bow. He invited me to call him Tim. He explained that his work was mainly with people who were depressed. I hadn't had much experience with this myself and confessed that I'd always felt uneasy around people with depression. 'Maybe that's because you've never dealt with your own', he quietly suggested. I was taken aback by his words, but they proved to be prophetic.

He asked me why I was uneasy around depressed people, and I explained that I saw them as angry people who had turned their anger on themselves. I feared they might turn it on me if I got too close. This was naïve on my part, but he seemed to take what I said very seriously. 'Maybe you could be of help to us', he said. 'It would be interesting to have you sit with our therapists during their live sessions to see if you can spot this anger and track how it is expressed.' I was touched: Tim Beck felt I could bring fresh thinking to his centre of excellence. He added just one proviso: I was to write out all the ways I expected to see depressed people being angry before I saw anyone.

After two weeks of sitting in on therapy sessions, I met Tim in his office to report on what I had observed. In the sessions I attended, I hadn't witnessed one person whose problem was inverted anger. I told Beck that all I had seen were people whose hearts were broken, usually in the wake of some loss, and struggling to come to terms with that loss. What surprised me was how each therapist I watched seemed to restore their client's confidence to deal with problems that were overwhelming them.

However, I still had difficulty grasping the concept of cognitive therapy. Tim explained that he had noticed how people who were depressed often thought about their lives in very unhelpful ways. Cognitive therapy was simply a way to make them aware of how they were thinking and, rather than simply assume their thoughts to be true, to instead investigate them.

'That's a little like what you had me do', I replied. 'Rather than tell me that my perceptions about depressed people were naïve, you had me make them explicit and then check them out.' Tim nodded; that was exactly what he'd been trying to do. Now I was ready to start training with him.

Beck was an exceptional psychotherapist. He had trained and practised as a psychoanalyst for over 20 years before he developed cognitive therapy. He knew his way around the unconscious and greatly respected how it shaped our thinking and behaviour. His analytic practice had given him a feel for what was unspoken in the therapy session, what lies just beyond the reach of the conscious mind.

I remember sitting with him one day when he saw a young man in his late twenties who had recently lost his job and his girlfriend. The young man was completely despondent. He sat crouched in the chair, his eyes welling up every few moments. He had no interest in engaging with life. He didn't know why he was seeing Beck and felt there was little point in him doing so. He was a loser, and Beck couldn't do anything about that. He asked Beck in a frustrated tone what he could offer. Tim spoke softly to him and said something like, 'I know what you're saying feels completely real. You believe it wholeheartedly. And it hurts like hell. But I'm also aware that a part of you got up and figured out how to make it here today for this appointment. It's the part of your mind that can think clearly. My job is to support that part of your mind so it can help the part of you that's hurting.'

Tim told me in later years that what he valued most about CBT were three core principles of the model that had nothing to do with negative thoughts. The first was collaboration. Beck was also uneasy with the power dynamics of the traditional 'expert vs patient' psychotherapy relationship. He preferred a more collaborative approach, where therapist and client worked as a team on specific issues the client identified as important.

The second principle of CBT he called 'guided discovery'. This was especially important to Beck. He insisted on the therapist being comfortable 'not knowing' everything in the client's mind and asking thoughtful questions to clarify things. For this approach to be most effective, the therapist needed to ask questions with genuine curiosity and openness to learning something new.

The third feature that Beck believed to be critical to the effectiveness of CBT was homework. This was of particular interest to me and became the focus of my PhD. Traditionally, therapies and treatments for mental health difficulties encouraged the people receiving them to be passive, to merely take the tablets, to simply show up to therapy sessions and talk. The assumption was that drugs would do most of the work of recovery, and insights gained in therapy would simply naturally translate into constructive changes in one's life. Psychologists and therapists have increasingly exposed such assumptions as untrue.

Homework encourages clients to confront particular aspects of their life away from the therapist's office, where they need to take initiative. Carefully planned assignments create opportunities for clients to confront their fears, complete tasks in a manageable way and investigate their assumptions about other people. The purpose of homework is to restore a person's sense of agency – their belief that they can make a difference. 'Action is a pre-condition of learning,' as the Swiss psychologist Jean Piaget wrote.[8] We can't think our way into a new way of living, but we can live our way into a new way of thinking.

Since then, CBT has been universally established as the most popular form of psychotherapy.

One reason for this is that CBT promotes itself as a 'time-limited' intervention. Originally, 12 sessions were considered ideal, but recent trends in oversubscribed mental health services have reduced the recommended course of CBT to six sessions. Current practice for most people admitted to in-patient psychiatric hospitals is a course of SSRI antidepressants and six sessions of CBT. This may be fine for some people, particularly if delivered skilfully. Unfortunately, follow-up research reports that many people receiving this combination relapse soon afterwards.[9]

My doctoral study investigated key variables that predicted compliance with homework and positive gains from therapy. One hundred and thirty-two therapists working in private healthcare settings across the USA participated, and they returned data on 348 CBT clients. The results highlighted the importance of the client's commitment to change, their belief that this approach could work for them, their level of hope that recovery was possible, and an emotionally attuned relationship between client and therapist.

One thing I found surprising was the number of CBT sessions these clients were undertaking – an average of over 30. One client had been attending consistently for over five years. This was clearly at odds with the number of sessions CBT proponents recommended. I considered that perhaps these longer-term clients had evidence of more complicated mental health issues, but data revealed this was not the case. Their scores on anxiety and depression tests were in the normal range. When I looked more closely at the client sample, I found them to be an educated, professional and resourceful group.

While in no way wanting to diminish the reality of these client's struggles or the value of the therapy being offered to them, I wondered whether this might be a true reflection of what happens in many psychotherapy centres where clients are welcome to attend for as long as they wish – provided they can afford to pay.

I asked Beck what he thought. He agreed that 12 sessions of CBT couldn't touch some of the deeper childhood issues that require a long time to surface and be safely processed. He also suggested that relationships with therapists can be invaluable to a person whose everyday life may lack trusted friends and allies. This led me to think about the social context of psychotherapy. One English psychologist, David Smail, argued that while psychotherapists proclaim to offer a scientifically-based technology of change, the reality is that they offer solace and acceptance. Cultural myths suggest that the possibility of contentment exists if only we can overcome our sadness, low self-esteem or anxiety. Many people's greatest frustration and sense of inadequacy results from their inevitable failure to achieve what the cultural myth tells them must be achieved. He wondered if, for some people, therapy could never end because the reality is that we all fall short of how adjusted, confident and successful we feel we should be. For others, therapy may be necessary as it offers an opportunity for genuine human contact where they feel accepted despite their vulnerabilities and failures.[10]

I returned from that first visit to the USA with a new skill that radically changed how I was perceived as a psychologist. I was also asked to teach others CBT. This led to several training courses until I established the MSc in Cognitive Psychotherapy at Trinity College Dublin in the mid-1990s.

CBT gets people back on their feet and helps them recover the confidence they need to face difficulties in their lives. The unexpected findings in my study, however, pointed me beyond the individual to the wider social and cultural context of mental pain. Mental health is not just an individual matter. We need to consider that people's negative thoughts may not only reflect how they see themselves. We need to look beyond a person's immediate social context and wonder about the influences on them by a culture that sets specific expectations for men and women and defines standards of behaviour that constitute good mental health.

5

THE BODY NEVER LIES

The body is the guardian of the truth, our truth,
because it carries the experience of a lifetime.[1]

ALICE MILLER

When I completed training and graduated with a Master's Degree in Applied Psychology, I was appointed basic grade clinical psychologist in St James's. This was the teaching hospital for the Department of Psychiatry at Trinity College. It was situated in the heart of Old Dublin and was run under the auspices of St Patrick's Hospital, a nearby private psychiatric service. St Pat's, as it is colloquially known, had been contracted to develop a community mental health service for inner city Dublin and some of its adjoining neighbourhoods. Hospital Six had 50 inpatient beds, a day hospital, several outlying community services and hostels.

My supervisor, Helen Haughton, was a gifted senior clinical psychologist who profoundly influenced me. An educated, well-spoken woman, she was both respected and feared in the corridors of St Pat's. She was a strong advocate for patients and their families and was frequently critical of what she regarded as the 'over-medicalisation' of their suffering. Despite the formalities observed among senior medical staff at the time, she could be forthright in her challenges. I remember one occasion, at a weekly case conference, where I sensed her mounting frustration as the significant losses a person had experienced were dismissed in favour of an exclusively biological explanation for his depression. She stood up, looked the medical director in the eye and said, 'Can you not see how bereaved this man is? Haven't you read anything about attachment theory?'

Psychotherapy training was patchy in Ireland in the 1980s. Mostly, mental health professionals invited teachers from abroad to conduct weekend workshops here on a monthly or bi-monthly basis. In 1983, I joined a group of psychologists who had created a longer, more in-depth training course in Gestalt therapy, a type of psychotherapy that emphasises self-awareness and focuses on the present moment rather than past experiences. A trainer from Germany visited every two months and conducted four-day workshops at a venue outside Belfast. There was some teaching, but for the most part, training required each of us to work on our issues in a group therapy setting.

During one of these workshops, I shared that I felt very lonely even as I sat there surrounded by other group members. I felt curiously distant from them all. Our leader, Marianne, asked me whether any image that described how I was feeling came into my mind. In my mind, it was as though there was a wall of glass between myself and the group.

Marianne invited me to stay with my experience. As I did, it became more and more oppressive. Suddenly, I imploded emotionally. My whole body crumpled as I fell to the ground. What followed were alternating outbursts of sobbing and rage. I crawled around on my hands and knees, pressing my face hard against the carpet. I had no idea what was happening to me but I allowed myself to just go with it. No one said a word or dared to intervene.

Later that evening, I wrote the following entry about the experience in my journal:

> I threw my body on the floor, sobbing, screeching, feeling enormous pain. Marianne asked me what I was feeling. 'Nobody can reach me' was my eventual reply. By the time I said this, I had squirmed halfway across the room; my face had been pushed down on the floor, my arms gripping the carpet as if to get the ground to open up and swallow me. I wanted to die. That was the only way that I could give up the struggle. I wanted something, some God, to take me and tell me that I had tried hard enough. That it was OK to stop. In death, I would find peace. I cried a lot and stayed down on the floor. Marianne spoke quietly as though to a child. I felt her powerful presence. She never interrupted, just echoed what I said to let me know I was being heard.

That felt good. At some point, I remember her saying how important it would be for God to take me on his knee and how my dad never had. That rang true. After a little more time had passed, she asked me what I wanted to do next. I couldn't answer; I just laughed and cried. I remained on the ground with my eyes shut as she allowed the group to take a break. I heard people move, but I didn't move. I lay there as people passed by. I felt the touch of caring hands. One person lay both hands on my head. But I was cut off from them as though trapped in some dark place.

I had no explanation for my outburst, but I recognised it was entirely out of character for me to be so dramatic. I wondered if I had had a re-experience of my birth. 'Rebirthing' was a popular intervention in psychotherapy in the 1980s. People were encouraged to relive their birth and release any residual tension they had experienced at that time. Perhaps I had a traumatic birth. I needed to find out the truth.

My mother was sitting in her favourite chair in the dining room when I arrived home that day. After the usual catch-up over a pot of tea, I asked she could help me clarify some things. 'Can you tell me something about my birth?' I asked. She described a quick, trouble-free delivery on a mid-summer morning. She needed no medical assistance and had been able to sit up with me from the beginning.

She was curious and asked me what had suddenly made this question important to me. With some reluctance, I told her about the incident at the training workshop. I only got as far as describing my experience of feeling cut off from everyone in the room, 'as though there was a pane of glass between me and everyone else,' when she started to cry. I didn't expect this. After a few moments, she said she had some idea about my experience. It was something in my childhood that she'd assumed I had forgotten entirely.

For the first time in my life, I heard the story of my admission to the Cork Fever Hospital. Her words poured out like she had needed to say them for years. But it was hard to hear and more information than I could handle. At some point, she paused, and I asked if we might leave it for now. She could see that I was rattled, and offered to write it all down so I could read about what happened at my own pace.

Over the next two months, my mother sent me several long letters, detailing with forensic precision what had happened to Jim and what had happened to me before, during and after discharge from the hospital. She bitterly regretted leaving me in Cork with her parents for so long after only a few weeks at home with her. But she couldn't cope. There was too much happening, and she had very little support.

My mother was an excellent writer. Every detail of her letters was a body blow. It took me days to get through each one of them. Some days one paragraph was as much as I could digest. Reading her words was more manageable than listening to her tell me in person, where I would have had to deal with her reactions as well as my own, but it was an ordeal. Maybe the truth sets us free, but it burns you up inside before it does.

I read her final letter the following September, just before I flew to the States for a five-year career break. I had a lot to process but needed to shelve it. I had to prioritise settling into a new job and finding a home for my family.

Attachment theory, and my mother's letters, helped me to understand my back story. It showed me that my life started well and that I felt loved and secure as an infant, but my hospitalisations and subsequent separations left me feeling abandoned. My mother's inability to stay with me as I worked through my feelings resulted in our fractured relationship. But she was isolated and vulnerable herself. She had little confidence in her own judgement and couldn't ask for the support she needed.

As an adult, these age-old insecurities could still be triggered by any loss of affection or respect. I quickly fell into self-blame. I assume this echoes a childhood survival strategy when blaming myself for feeling bad was probably much easier than blaming my parents. But these insecurities, when inflamed, could also trigger episodes of depression.

A great deal of human suffering is packed into the single word 'depression'. The sorrow we feel when we lose someone we love, the deep hurt we feel when we are betrayed, and the helplessness we feel when we are trapped in an oppressive situation where there is no way out. We fall into a dark place where we are lost to ourselves. Our bodies fill with pain until we almost suffocate. We are drained of energy; sleep gives us little or no reprieve. Our minds turn against us. We are 'losers'; we always have been and always will be.

I've been deeply depressed several times, and it took me years to understand why. But even when I did, the depression didn't stop happening. Finding my way through depression has come from long stretches where I was trapped inside it.

My most painful experience of depression hit me at a time when everything looked optimal in my life. In 1985, I was offered a five-year work contract at the University of Pennsylvania from 1985 to 1990. During that visit, I would ultimately become licensed as a clinical psychologist and complete my PhD research. By any account, this was a major career opportunity and promised an adventure that would be good for all my family. But I had barely unpacked my bags when I was plunged into a darkness that lasted almost two years.

6

THINGS FALL APART

Things fall apart; the centre cannot hold[1]

WILLIAM BUTLER YEATS

n September 1985, having accepted the job offer, I arranged
a leave of absence from St James's Hospital and headed to
the USA. I travelled ahead of my family to find a place for us
to live. Leaving Ursula, Andrew, Philip and our six-month-
old daughter Rachel wasn't easy, but it was necessary.

The work situation I found waiting for me was more
fraught than I'd expected. There was a lot of tension among
my new colleagues. Any illusions that I would be welcomed
with open arms were quickly shattered.

Having previously spent a year in Philadelphia in 1981, I was
familiar with its various neighbourhoods and decided to look
for a home in Narberth. This safe, old-world neighbourhood
had a good public school, an old-style cinema, a launderette,
a bar and a small grocery store. Within a week or two, I found
a three-bed house for sale and arranged to view it. The house
was on Conway Ave, a block from the village centre. It was a

stand-alone two-storey property with a basement, a porch and a garden, front and back. It backed onto a neighbourhood park with a playground and a Little League baseball pitch. Next door to the house was a quaint fire station. The house was near the end of the avenue and beside a train line. The station where I would catch a commuter train to work was a hundred yards away. A school bus stopped at the end of this avenue every morning to take children to the local public school. We were unlikely to find a safer and more convenient place to live.

The asking price was affordable, and a mortgage was readily available. I wrote a cheque for two thousand dollars to cover the booking deposit and gave it to the agent. The house was mine.

However, my good news was greeted with alarm by my work colleagues. 'No one buys the first house they see; there are probably better deals out there,' exclaimed one.

'What do you mean it's beside a fire station? Do you know how loud fire trucks can be?' said another. They warned me that I would be woken up by screaming sirens or the rattle of passing trains. The more I listened, the more convinced I became that I had acted impulsively and foolishly. Feeling nauseous, I realised my family would pay the price for my poor judgement.

I needed to make things right. I revisited the realtor before things went any further. Back in her office two days later, I asked her to return my cheque. She was a patient lady and genuinely concerned for me. She returned my cheque but encouraged me to take my time and think about things. This was a well-minded home, in very good repair, on a quiet avenue, within my price range. In her view, the noise would not be an issue as the fire station had only a single fire truck manned by a volunteer crew who rarely got called out. And the nearby tracks served a fleet of electrified commuter trains which purred noiselessly along and rarely at night.

But my mind was already crowded with images of living in a tiny, cramped house where our sleep would be disrupted by the shrill of passing trains and screaming sirens. I couldn't hear what she was saying. I tore up the cheque I was holding in my hands.

In the days that followed, I felt relief. My colleagues congratulated me for being proactive and not allowing myself to be duped into purchasing a property I would regret forever. Several weeks later, I found a more spacious rental property in Narberth.

In early December, I drove to JFK Airport in New York to pick up my family and bring them to what would be home for all of us for the foreseeable future. I stood at the arrival gate until they appeared. Ursula was carrying Rachel on her back and wheeling a trolley loaded with suitcases; the boys were carrying their bags beside her.

It had been three months since we'd been together. I only realised how much I'd missed them when we wrapped our arms around each other. Andrew greeted me with a big smile and a warm, 'Hi, Dad.' Philip walked up to me and kicked my leg, probably a more honest emotional reaction to his dad being AWOL for three months. Rachel beamed at me from the carrier on her mother's back but had no idea who this stranger was.

It was late and we were exhausted when we arrived back in Narberth. We all went to bed. The next day I showed them the house and drove them around the neighbourhood.

I told Ursula about my near-disaster with Conway Ave. She was sorry it had been such an ordeal for me. In hindsight, she felt that being apart had made everything more stressful than it needed to be, as we had always made such big decisions together. As we toured Narberth, she asked me to show her the house on Conway Ave. I hadn't been there since the night the estate agent showed me around.

It was a bright, clear December day as we turned into the avenue. The house that I nearly bought looked more substantial than I remembered. The street was lined on both sides with well-kept homes. Firemen were polishing an antique fire engine straight out of 'Fireman Tom'. Families were playing in the park behind the house. Everything looked idyllic. This unsettled me. Ursula commented, 'What a beautiful street and lovely house; we'd have been fine living here.'

That's when I saw it. I'd allowed a gift to slip through my fingers. I'd been anxious, ungrounded and too easily swayed by others' opinions. A cold chill crept over me, and a sickening feeling rose in my stomach. Something broke inside me.

We all have mini-breakdowns. Moments when we lose our bearings, feel terrified, tormented, confused by what's happening to us and unsure what to do next. These painful moments are part of the intensity of being human. They're not necessarily a bad thing. They stop us in our tracks and may make us realise that we've been missing something, deceiving ourselves, hurting others intentionally or unintentionally, or refusing to accept that some goal we are stubbornly pursuing is not working. They're uncomfortable and disconcerting, certainly. But these moments can prompt us to make important course corrections.

Breakdowns that persist over an extended period are something else, however. These are what we are usually referring to when we talk about 'mental health vulnerabilities'. Emotional difficulties from the past merge with the problems we are facing in the present and weigh heavily on our hearts. Our lives feel overwhelming. The future is impossible to see through the thick mental fog that falls over us.

The realisation of my foolishness regarding Conway Avenue shouldn't have been as upsetting or painful as it proved. I hadn't ever owned it. I had taken advice from bright, experienced adults who knew the market better than I ever would. But it had broken me in a way I hadn't ever experienced before. It was like it kicked open some door where everything bad in my life had been hidden. And I felt I would never be able to close that door again.

In the weeks and months that followed, I went through the motions of a functioning adult. I performed dad duties and related as best I could to family and friends. I kept my distance from colleagues and feigned empathy with clients at work. Many of them didn't seem nearly as miserable as I was. And when they were, all I could say was, 'I know exactly how you feel.'

I put in eight-hour work days, but on my way home, I had nothing left. I turned my face into the window of the commuter train, acknowledged the full force of my pent-up pain and wept. My body ached, my emotions felt dark and heavy, and my mind was full of cruel accusations.

I hated being depressed. I did everything I could to kill the pain. But it followed me relentlessly. I recall one morning I went running early because I couldn't sleep. I couldn't shake off the darkness no matter how fast I ran. I felt frustrated and angry. When I returned to our street, I stopped by a tall stone wall at the end of our road. Without thinking, I started to bang my head lightly against it. It hurt, but I also felt some welcome relief. The reprieve was short-lived, so I hit the wall harder each time. I wanted to close down my mind. I only stopped when I noticed blood running down my face.

Being around my family became unbearable. My inability to engage with them constantly reminded me what a worthless person I was. By late January, I had moved into the attic. I disappeared up there when the children had gone to bed. Then I drank beer and smoked until I fell asleep on an old double mattress some former tenant had abandoned.

I clung to self-deception rather than admit to myself or anyone else how bad things were. Because all I could think about was my pain, I completely missed how hurtful and selfish my behaviour seemed to others. On 28 February, Rachel's first birthday, I sat at the kitchen table and stared as Ursula lit the single candle on the cake. I couldn't feel a thing.

That was the last straw for Ursula. She'd been urging me to get help, but I was frightened that if I did, I would lose whatever semblance of control I had. Instead, I focused on keeping my job and looking after my family economically. But she couldn't take anymore. She packed the children onto a train and headed to Washington, DC, to stay with a friend. She would return when I'd decided to get help.

And that's how I found myself sitting in an office in early March, waiting to see someone who could help. I didn't feel hopeful. The psychologist I had arranged an appointment with was Dr Doug Schoeninger. When he stepped into the room, I saw a tall, handsome man with a kind face. He greeted me warmly. That helped.

After gathering the usual biographical details, he asked me, 'How are you doing?' There was so much I could have said in response to his enquiry, but what came to me then was, 'I'm worried that I'm turning into my dad'. I told him I had an image from my childhood of my dad spending evenings sitting in his chair in the dining room corner, watching TV, smoking and drinking into the late hours. I had brought a

13-inch portable TV into the attic and was recreating all his mannerisms. Doug responded, 'When we're stressed, we go home'. I knew then that I was in the right place.

Home was a recurring motif of my depression. Being separated from home, searching for a home, and finding and losing a home appeared to have been a catalyst for my downfall. Before Ursula and the children joined me, I had felt unmoored. Being reunited with them should have grounded me and lifted my mood. For some reason, it hadn't. If anything, it made me feel worse. My retreat to the attic may have been a radical attempt to re-create what, for me, represented home.

I told Doug what a miserable husband and father I was. But I couldn't translate my remorse into meaningful action. His responses let me gradually take responsibility for my behaviour without reinforcing my shame.

Psychotherapy is marketed today as a time-limited, brief affair. Sometimes, that can be enough. But complex emotional wounds that we've carried in our bodies for years take time to resolve. My 'real estate crisis' wasn't just about losing a place to live but about a library of losses and insecurities that finally caught up with me. It also precipitated a crisis of trust in my judgement. If I'd got it wrong about a simple house purchase, how could I ever trust my judgement again in my personal and professional life?

Recovery isn't straightforward; one day, we step into the light, and the next, we double back into darkness. There were days when Doug and I made significant breakthroughs that gave me a taste of peace with myself. But those moments of liberation were often followed by the return of gut-wrenching pain that made little sense. My depression was a painful experience, but it was an experience that invited me, even demanded of me, to grow up. It was not the 'black dog' that Winston Churchill had described; it was a 'guide dog' that mapped my path to becoming more real. In this sense, I could not dismiss it as an anomaly in my brain, a chemical balance that simply needed to be rebalanced.

I believed that my depression had a lot to do with my early life, and I knew that I needed the help of my family to understand why I was feeling as poorly as I did. Family therapy was perhaps a rather formal way to go about this, but it would provide a safe space where each of us would have a chance to say whatever we needed. I hoped that our sessions would also include a conversation about Jim. After all, his life and death had remained our best-kept secret for a long time.

And so, in 1986, I wrote to my parents and spoke candidly about how I felt. I received a beautiful reply from my dad, who empathised with me as much as any army officer could and offered to do anything he could to help. I asked them if he and my mum would consider coming to the States to join me in some therapy sessions. It was a big ask, but they agreed to come for an extended visit and do whatever it took to get me back on my feet.

At our first session, my mother looked at my father and asked through tears, 'How did Jim die?' She was finally able to ask, thirty years after her son had been buried. Dad explained, as best he could, the medical reasons for his death. He reassured her that Jim didn't suffer and how he would have been chronically brain-damaged, 'a vegetable', in his words, had he lived. 'All in all,' he said, 'We were all better off, including Jim.' A strategic military assessment, no doubt, that failed to recognise the trauma his death had been for all of us, himself included. But at least we were finally talking about Jim.

In the course of our sessions, we also discussed many other aspects of my childhood that had been a puzzle to me, and we spoke about what we did well and not so well as a family. At one point, in an attempt to lighten the atmosphere, I jokingly said, 'Well, this is good; Oedipus can finally retire.'

I was smiling, but my mother was frowning. 'I know,' she said. 'It wasn't fair, but even at four, you understood me better than your father.' Her admission jolted me, but there was some truth in what she said. I'd always been able to sense her moods. I heard her crying in her bedroom. She fought so hard to keep everything inside, and mostly she kept her pain well hidden. But when she couldn't conceal it anymore, her behaviour became confusing, sometimes terrifying. I remember watching her come down the stairs one Sunday afternoon. Her eyes were red, and she was carrying a small suitcase. As she opened the front door, she said she 'couldn't take any more' and walked out the front gate. Neither my siblings nor I knew what she meant. Standing inside the sitting room window looking at her walk away, I felt it was somehow my fault. She returned a few hours later as I put together something for tea.

My mother explained that she'd grown up hearing the mantra, 'Not a word'. Not a word about her own mother's depression, not a word about her father's alcoholism, not a word about how upset she might feel in herself. She had adopted this creed and always tried to conceal her pain. But not anymore. Finally, my mum spoke openly about her feelings and promised that from now on, she would always do so. While it was hard to hear the full extent of how distressed she had been, her honesty lifted some of the burden of guilt I'd been carrying for way too long.

In our final family therapy session, we returned to Jim. We would all be together that May for his anniversary. We discussed how best to commemorate his short life and how we might 'let him go'. Doing this would involve the help and support of some people with whom we had formed an important friendship in Philadelphia. But it would also require facing up to the truth of the events that had followed Jim's death, and some very hard truths about Ireland.

7

LET US NOT TALK FALSELY NOW

fter Jim's death, life in our house had moved on. Two new brothers and a baby sister arrived, and my parents became consumed by the challenges every young family faces. But no mother forgets the death of a son. Every year, she would take us on a bus to Deansgrange Cemetery, many miles from northside Dublin. She was convinced that Jim's remains were there. My siblings and I would stand in silence opposite the 'Angels' plot' and say a prayer for him. It was 30 years before I learned the truth – and it was revealed by chance in a surprising remark from my father.

When our second son, Philip, was a year old, Ursula and I bought a house off the South Circular Road. It was a terraced house with no side or rear entrance. On moving day, every item of furniture had to be carried through the front door. My father and I took my two little boys to a nearby park to make things easier for our movers and helpers.

Harold's Cross has a triangular-shaped park with a small playground. While the boys played, my father and I stood watching the children and chatting. At some point in the conversation, he pointed to the high wall surrounding Mount Jerome Cemetery directly across the road and said, 'That's where Jim was buried?' At first, I had no idea what he was talking about. When I finally grasped the implications of what he was saying, I thought he must have been confused. I reminded him that Jim was buried in the 'Angels' plot' in Deansgrange Cemetery; he'd been well aware of our mother's annual pilgrimages.

And that's when I heard the story of Jim's death, Dad's journey to Mount Jerome cemetery with Jim's little white coffin and how he left the coffin in the shade of a tree. He had never told my mother because he didn't want to upset her. It was enough that she had lost her child; no need to make it any worse. I also sensed that he wasn't too proud of deserting his son's remains in an empty graveyard and had wanted to put the whole affair behind him.

Nothing more was said about the matter for several months. But Ursula decided to investigate whether Mount Jerome had any record of Jim. She had grown up in rural Ireland where her family had a funeral business. Visiting graves was a routine part of everyday life. It seemed natural to her that we should locate Jim's grave so that our family could visit it. When passing the cemetery one day, she decided to ask the caretaker if this would be possible.

Ursula stepped into the cemetery's main office. She met a man there who consulted a series of thick ledgers to conduct a grave search. They kept meticulous records. Because she had a name and a date, he was able to identify a plot number and show her where Jim was buried on a large map.

He walked with her to the northwestern tip of the cemetery and pointed out an unmarked scrap of dirt. He explained to her that this insignificant-looking plot had served as a burial site for St Patrick's Mother and Baby Home on the Navan Road. Jim had been buried in a grave for 'unwanted children'.

Children from St Patrick's were usually buried in the Angels' Plot at Glasnevin Cemetery, but some children, usually those considered 'unwanted', were interred in Mount Jerome. These were children that no one had cared to bury ceremonially. Jim was not alone. The caretaker believed there could be up to a hundred babies under that patch of dirt.

I remembered St Patrick's well. It was close to where we lived in Villa Park, and I'd walked past it regularly. It had operated for 81 years as an institution for 'unmarried' mothers and their 'illegitimate' babies. It was the largest of Ireland's nine mother-and-baby homes, providing up to 149 beds for mothers and 560 places for children. A 2021 state-commissioned report on mother and baby homes revealed appalling conditions in St Patrick's. Specifically, it detailed overcrowding, poor facilities, criminal lack of medical training in antenatal care, and an alarmingly high infant mortality rate. At some unknown point in time, Saint Patrick's also established a 'secure unit' for women who returned pregnant a second time. They were known as 'repeat offenders', and their area was off-limits to the first-time 'offenders'. Other mother and baby homes usually refused 'second-timers', and they were sent instead to Saint Patrick's.

Historical records show infant mortality at St Patrick's was up to 50 per cent when the national rate was just 6 per cent or 7 per cent. Outbreaks of infection spread rapidly in overcrowded and cramped conditions. Survivors described regular physical, psychological and sexual abuse. Mixed-race babies and children were beaten, abused and shamed throughout their care. These children were rarely adopted and were typically moved to industrial schools, such as the Artane Industrial School for Boys, once they were old enough. Here they experienced an even greater level of abuse and neglect. The Daughters of Charity, the Catholic nuns who ran St Patrick's, recently apologised for the trauma experienced by mothers and babies under their care: 'We regret that we could not have done more to ease the burden and suffering carried by these women.'

However tragic Jim's death was for our family, uncovering the details of his death reminded us of a much darker story of infant neglect and mortality.

Having located Jim's grave, we could formally lay him to rest and restore his place in the wider family. But our unfinished business was postponed when I received the job offer from the University of Pennsylvania and began the process of moving and settling my family into our home there. We invited my parents to visit and in the spring of 1986, they came and stayed for two months. Now, 31 years later, my parents and I finally talked about Jim. We could, at last, explore ways to meaningfully remember him.

A small community of nuns lived in an old red-brick house a street away from our rental home in West Philly. They were active in the neighbourhood, teaching in the local community school and befriending the most vulnerable through various social services. Their home provided a sanctuary for struggling people in many different ways. When we first visited the States in 1981, they had taken us in as a family. Sr Dorothy taught Andrew to play chess, and Sr Sheila often babysat for us. When we returned to the States in 1985, we picked up our friendship with that community of nuns.

They had turned one room in their home into a small chapel. We knew this would be the perfect place for Jim's memorial.

We invited another friend of ours, Irish-American Jesuit, Fr Nick Rashford, to be the celebrant. The day we picked for the memorial was May 16th, the day Jim died. When the morning arrived, we were silently concerned for each other. We knew it would be an emotional day, and we didn't want it to overwhelm any of us.

Dad took care of the logistics: Where were the car keys? Where were the tissues? Was there film in the camera? He would use this as a prop to hide behind later. We climbed into our Pontiac and headed into West Philly.

My parents, family and our hosts sat in a half-circle on fold-out chairs. Nick welcomed us by name and spoke in a reassuring way. He said we were there to remember someone we'd loved because he'd been very important to us. The familiar cadence of Mass helped to settle us.

My mother had brought a framed black and white photograph she'd kept hidden for years. It was a photo of Jim and me. Three weeks before his death, she had taken refuge from the rain with us in a doorway on Westmorland Street. Noticing a sign inside the door that advertised a photographer upstairs, she carried us both up to his studio and had our picture taken. This was somewhat reckless because money was scarce. But she didn't have a photo of us and wanted one. We placed that photograph on the small altar.

Our daughter, Rachel, barely two years old, wandered behind the altar. Father Nick invited her to stand beside him. He also beckoned Andrew and Philip to do the same. Standing as far back as possible in that small space, my father lifted the camera and captured the moment.

Towards the end of Mass, Nick gave us a chance to say anything we wanted to say. We shared a few moments of silence in his memory. And then we let him go and wished him well. The tears came. I hugged my mother for the first time in decades and felt her arms around me. After several decades of strain and distance, it was unfamiliar but comforting. She said, 'I feel like I've just lost two stone in weight.'

When my parents returned to Dublin, they did something brave and creative. They visited Mount Jerome Cemetery and negotiated the purchase of the mass grave where Jim was buried. It took some persuasion, and only when they'd signed over their rights to bury anyone else were they allowed to buy the plot.

They wanted to erect a headstone. My father had the idea of including a blessing, 'For all those interred within', carved into the border surrounding the grave. All these children had been laid in this unmarked ground. Over the years, they and the mothers who bore them were forgotten, with no one to tell their stories. I've often wondered about the grief of those who gave birth to them. I wonder who decided that they were 'unwanted'? I imagine many of those mothers had loved their children no less than my mother loved Jim.

In contrast to Jim, who was cherished in every moment of his brief life, what happened to those children is hard to contemplate. The treatment of those who lived and died in our state institutions reveals a shadow side to the Irish psyche we'd rather deny. While we might wish that all of what happened could be laid at the doors of religious orders, the truth is that we were all implicated to some extent. We turned a blind eye, many of us knowing all was not right inside the walls of those institutions but saying nothing out of deference to authorities in whom we placed our trust.

In his book, *The Best Catholics in the World,* a historical account of institutional abuse in Ireland, Irish journalist Derek Scally wrote that 'for many Irish bystanders, their ongoing, deep silence is the silence of people with nowhere to go with their memories and their conflicted feelings.'[1]

My family and I were among those bystanders. We moved from the Navan Road to the Malahide Road when I was seven. The now infamous Artane Industrial School for Boys was on the same road. On Sunday afternoons, we watched boys walk in single file along the high wall of the O'Brien Institute, which faced our home; an unbroken line of children moving slowly behind a lone Christian brother who led the way. To my young eyes, they looked 'odd'. Maybe because they were dressed in shabby clothes, either too big or too small for them, maybe because they weren't talking. They looked more like a chain gang of convicts being moved from one location to another rather than a group of children on a day out.

I remember one sunny Sunday afternoon when they passed in front of our house. All of us were out in the front garden. We stopped whatever we were doing to look over at them. My mother reminded us all how 'lucky' those boys were: 'Nobody wanted them. If it weren't for the Christian Brothers looking after them, they'd have no one.'

Even then, her words were confusing. I grew up in Artane's shadow, whose reputation inspired fear and trembling. We didn't know what went on behind those walls, except that the boys had to work hard and got beaten if they stepped out of line. If we were ever 'bold' at home or school, we were threatened with admission to Artane.

Years later, as a psychologist in St James's Hospital, I met several Artane survivors who were older adults by then. I'd been asked to write a psychological report on the impact of growing up in Artane on their mental health. Long-term trauma was suspected in many who had been there as children. Their collective experiences were the subject of a Commission established to investigate child abuse within institutions in Ireland. The eventual report, published in 2009, comprised seven volumes and became known as the Ryan Report.

The men I saw lived in inner-city Dublin within the catchment area of St. James's Hospital. Most of them lived alone in Dublin Corporation flats. What I listened to was more horrific than anything I'd heard or imagined previously. The sexual aspects of the abuse they experienced were just one part of the even darker ordeals they endured for years. These men had been targeted as young children because there was only a minimal chance that they would ever be visited or that anyone might be interested in their welfare. In most cases, they had been sent there by families who lived 'down the country' or from other institutions, including St Patrick's on the Navan Road. These children were singled out and terrorised, sometimes on a nightly basis. They were taken from their dormitory stalls on the pretext that they had wet their beds or woken other boys with their crying. The sexual abuse they experienced was extreme.

Derek Scally recognises how much we want to avoid thinking about these things, that the 'sheer volume of horrors revealed have impaired our ability to reflect on what it was in Irish society that made these horrors possible'. But there comes a time when we must reflect if we are to come to terms with the subtle and not-so-subtle ways that these horrors still impact us. We don't come to terms with past wounds by forgetting they happened. Selective amnesia only heightens our chances of inadvertently re-enacting these traumas in each new generation.

In her study of intergenerational trauma passed down through generations in Ireland, Geraldine Moane in UCD wrote:

> One of the legacies of a history of oppression is … avoidance of pain, spiritual impoverishment and disconnection with self. These are the mechanisms underlying substance use commonly discussed in writings on oppression. This is an obvious area where a pattern that may have developed as an understandable response to oppression becomes embedded at cultural, family and psychological levels, transmitted over generations through intergenerational and cultural reproduction.[2]

I was part of a society that visited the atrocities of past generations on men, women and children throughout the twentieth century. Many of the religious orders who perpetuated abuse had themselves been brutalised and abused in their upbringing. We were part of a culture that implicitly condoned violence against children. We believed the thousands of people committed to psychiatric asylums were there because they needed to be. We believed the young women in the Magdalene Laundries were fortunate to have a roof over their heads and food on the table. Fearful of authority figures, especially religious authorities, we showed them undue deference. With very little awareness that we were doing so, we became silent witnesses to the inhumane treatment of our most vulnerable and innocent people.

If my own family experience concerning Jim's death taught me anything, it was that we need to come to terms with our past – we need to feel it, to talk about it honestly – if we are to stop carrying over the hurt and harm we experienced into our present and our future.

I visit Jim's grave every May. As brief as our shared life was, I've never doubted we were close. That bond has grown over the years. Sometimes, standing there, I cry. I miss him, but not as a sixteen-month-old child. I miss his friendship over the years, the person he might have married, the children they might have had, and the worlds we might have opened up to each other. My grief is not only for my baby brother, who was my companion for only 16 months, but for the person he would have become.

Over the next two years, my psyche became steadier. Gradually, I re-engaged with my family and made a serious effort to be a dad. Work settled into a manageable rhythm, and I no longer cried on the train home.

Close friends came to visit us and explore parts of the States. When they learned of my emotional struggles, they were genuinely concerned. Nobody could understand how losing a house – which had never actually been mine to lose – was such a heartache. They invariably tried to reassure me that I had dodged a bullet. One visitor even walked by the house on Conway Avenue and reported that he'd gotten a 'very bad feeling'. They tried to reassure me that what I had experienced as a loss was in reality a blessing. I've no doubt they had the best of intentions. But what struck me was their obvious discomfort with my pain. It's hard to see someone we care about suffer, but there are rarely easy answers for why we feel the way we do.

Therapists can be as guilty as anyone else in wanting to eliminate pain rather than listen to what it may be trying to communicate. They may reach for their preferred technique too early and too eagerly. When I directed the MSc in Cognitive Psychotherapy at Trinity College, Dublin, I annoyed students by repeatedly telling them to 'Stop trying to *help* people'. Rather than have them employ techniques to 'take out' unwanted thoughts, feelings and behaviours, I encouraged them to first and foremost be present and listen carefully to people's pain. The lesson I tried to teach was that a therapist might have as great an impact through their presence as they do through problem solving. Moments of insight usually happen in moments of silence a therapist allows within the session. A person may need to be alone in the safe presence of another to feel their feelings, as painful as they may be, without that person trying to 'help' them.

The person who did me the most good with respect to my crisis was someone who did exactly the opposite to everyone else. Eileen was an Irish-American social worker with a big heart. In her eyes, the world was wonderful, and being alive was the greatest gift of all. Even if her vision seemed somewhat rose-tinted to me, her joy was contagious. The world needed people like Eileen.

One summer night in 1987, after she spent the evening babysitting our children, I was driving Eileen home when she asked me how I was. I was about to launch into my usual reply – 'Everything is fine, thanks' – but stopped myself. There was something in her tone that called for honesty. I told her the whole saga of my loss and how it triggered a painful and protracted experience of depression for me. She never interrupted. Parked there on the sidewalk, I felt her silent presence. And I heard myself saying aloud, as if for the first time, how hurt I was by all that happened around that time, and the wounds it opened in me.

When I finished, she remained quiet. And then she said, with a lot of emotional conviction, 'What a horrible thing to happen. How could anyone ever get over such a loss?' Her words were simple and genuine. And as she spoke, I felt something inside me relax. Somebody finally got it. It had been incredibly tough for me to shake off that loss because so many other losses were folded into it. I no longer felt so bad for being stuck. Eileen's radical acceptance of my experience allowed me to own the experience, to feel OK about feeling as I did, and almost in the same breath, to put down this burden and move on with my life.

I barely noticed my depression lifting. Then one morning, shortly after I spoke with Eileen, I seemed to wake up as if I'd been asleep for the previous two years. I was driving through Fairmount Park into Philadelphia's city centre, my arm resting on the open window of my 12-year-old Pontiac. I felt a sensation on my face that I didn't recognise. For a moment, I was troubled. And then it dawned on me. I was feeling the breeze playing on my skin. It had been a long time since I had noticed such a sensation. At that same moment, it also hit me that my mood had been untroubled for the entire previous week. When I described the experience later to Ursula, she remarked, 'Sounds like what some people call normal.'

The psychoanalyst Wilfred Bion wrote, 'The mind grows through exposure to the truth.' He observed that mental health difficulties always involve resistance to the truth: 'A big part of what people want is evasion – evasion of regret, pain, guilt. As long as we evade truth, we create barriers to reality, particularly our psychic reality.'[3]

Our ability to face the truth varies according to how threatened or safe we feel. Sometimes the best we can do is to shut off our pain, keep our head down, and put one foot in front of the other. Dissociation can be vital to our survival. But our defences become problematic when we rely on them exclusively.

The mind needs truth the way a plant needs water; the mind that turns away from reality is in trouble. Life will always offer us moments to feel and express our truth. Moments of personal growth invariably follow some emotional crisis where denial is no longer an option. What looks like a breakdown to the unschooled eye may reflect the integration of experiences we have disowned. As we learn to befriend these feelings, we slowly come to terms with them and develop a fuller sense of identity. And we can be surprised to discover that we can bear them after years of being convinced they would break us.

THOUGHTS ABOUT THERAPY

Psychotherapy is concerned with the problems that people have in living their lives and in living with each other. The justification for psychotherapy is change – change in the aspect of life that has the potential to be under one's control.[1]

MARK AVELINE

Psychotherapy is a particular form of intimacy designed to enable someone to become more fully themselves. Groups and families may be the setting for therapy, but mainly it involves two people meeting and talking with each other in the hope that one of them can resolve distressing personal issues. Sometimes the source of their misery is known, but more than that person can handle. Their anguish may also be a mystery to them. All they know is that they have repeatedly been hitting the same wall and feel confused and demoralised. Therapy brings language, understanding and compassion to deep-seated wounds that keep us tethered to the past.

The quality of the therapeutic relationship is most important. It is the context in which change can happen.

Being seen and understood can empower a person to grow in precisely those places where they feel they can't develop further. This privileged relationship must be firmly grounded in a code of ethics that protects both parties.

Reminding therapists of what is expected of them, the psychoanalyst Nina Coltart wrote:

> It is required of us that we endure, understand, and help to change some extremes of emotion and fantasy in our patients; that we use our relationship with them to create greater insight between the patient and ourselves; that we do not exploit his or her dependence on us, emotionally, intellectually, sexually, or financially; that we assess when and how to draw the treatment to an appropriate close, and that we facilitate the patient's leaving us as completely as possible.[2]

For the person seeking help, therapy requires a series of risks, beginning with entering the unfamiliar world of the therapeutic relationship. Personal experiences that may never have been spoken of previously will need to be disclosed. Current and historical sources of distress need to be acknowledged and worked through emotionally. While a person wants relief, the path to recovery involves risk. It can take time before they trust their therapist with certain truths.

Recovery is always hard-won. Progress is never straightforward. It takes time for a person to feel confident enough to take responsibility for aspects of their problems that are potentially within their control, to risk relating to others in new ways and to make choices about how they want to live.

A not-so-good therapist has a plan for every new person before they walk in the door. They believe their pet theory will highlight whatever is amiss, and their therapeutic toolbox holds whatever techniques are required. Beware of such therapists; their narcissism blinds them. They are more committed to reinforcing their particular point of view than respecting the uniqueness of *this* person's difficulties.

A good therapist is comfortable with 'not knowing'. Each new person they meet is someone with problems they do not yet understand, whose symptoms mean something they have yet to grasp. Their 'not knowing' does not reflect their competence as a psychotherapist but is, instead, a mark of respect for the task ahead. Mental and emotional pain is complicated. If it were otherwise, the client would have sorted out their problems for themselves.

The therapist needs to listen. To discover how the person sitting before them is experiencing his or her world. And, through their attentive listening, to enable that person to listen to themselves. The more they both understand, the more they can see a way forward.

The terms 'being held' and 'contained' are often used to describe the experience of feeling safe and supported in the therapy relationship. The British child psychoanalyst, Donald Winnicott, observed that children flourished with mothers who provided a 'holding' or 'facilitating environment' for them and didn't needlessly interrupt their play. Winnicott believed that these same qualities applied to good psychotherapy. The therapist needs to 'hold' the client (in a non-physical way) and respect their capacity to find solutions for themselves. Another British psychoanalyst and writer, Wilfred Bion, similarly felt that, rather than solve a person's problems, the therapeutic relationship should enable them to reach new levels of understanding about their lives and draw on their resources. Both therapists believed that becoming oneself is more important than receiving knowledge, which can easily undermine a person's resourcefulness. As Winnicott wrote, 'The patient's creativity can only too easily be stolen by a therapist who knows too much.'[3]

Sitting quietly with intense emotion can be hard for a therapist. They may feel compelled to drop in some kind of 'explanation' or advice to reassure themselves that they have something to offer. But what is interesting is what can come to a therapist if they can 'hold' the space and sit with silence.

In a session one day with a woman who had been badly abused, both physically and sexually, she suddenly blurted out, 'I made him do it.' We'd been seeing one another for some time, but this was the dark secret she'd kept hidden for years. It seemed to come out of nowhere. It was unreasonable and completely untrue, and my first instinct was to reassure her that such an idea was outrageous. But it had taken a long time for her to say this 'out loud'. So, I sat with her in silence for a few moments. And after a while, I said what came to me in that silence: 'That's a very heavy burden to carry, and you've been carrying that for a long time.'

It can be frustrating for clients when the therapist doesn't jump in with a neat interpretation or some useful advice. I remember feeling furious with my lack of progress after a lengthy period of therapy. I was more unsure of what to do with my life than when we started. I pleaded with Ann, my therapist: 'I used to be a functioning human being. I used to be able to deal with stuff. Now, I'm a wreck. I don't think this process is doing me any good. Can we just cut to the chase? You know me, I've always been honest with you. Just tell me three things I should do. I promise you, whatever they are, I'll do them. I need to stop this and get back to living my life.'

She said nothing. Despite my heartfelt outburst, Ann was much too good a therapist to give in to my demands. I was in a very uncomfortable place. But she wasn't going to rescue me. Her silence invited me to move closer to whatever was happening inside me rather than distracting myself with the fantasy of being shown an easy way out. She didn't offer 'reassurance'.

Different therapists have different theories of what helps a person to change. Some theories highlight the importance of exploring early experiences which remain unresolved. Some believe that blocked emotions hold us back, and so encourage their expression and release. Other theories focus on how we think about ourselves and the world and highlight the need to identify blind spots and prejudices and actively challenge them.[4]

In contrast, other theories propose that the purpose of psychotherapy is to enable a conversation with and among a person's inner community of selves.[5] Existential psychotherapists such as Irving Yalom emphasise our capacity and responsibility to choose how we want to live in the present. We cannot change our past and must deal with whatever circumstances we face today. More recently, newer therapies – such as bioenergetic and sensorimotor therapy – have highlighted the need to undo various ways we hold tension and pain in the body. For example, Bessel van der Kolk, in his book *The Body Keeps the Score,* highlights how trauma is carried in the body and has a lasting impact on our lives, shaping every aspect of how we engage with the world:

> Traumatised people chronically feel unsafe inside their bodies: The past is alive in the form of gnawing interior discomfort. Their bodies are constantly bombarded by visceral warning signs. In an attempt to control these processes, they often become experts at ignoring their gut feelings and in numbing awareness of what is playing out inside. They learn to hide from themselves.[6]

Humans have an immense talent for expressing and making sense of their experiences through language. But in therapy, much of what is happening is non-verbal. It may be a long time before hurt that has never before been articulated can be processed in words. Many memories are not encoded as words at all but as body memories. Experiences of shock, abuse, confusion and loss are often carried in the body as sensations, behavioural patterns and particular postures. Paying attention to a person's body language can tell us a lot about what someone is struggling to express. Movement, role-play and particular body-based exercises can help release blocked energies. Finding the right words can be frustrating as they fall far short of expressing a person's inner tensions and sensations. As Suzanne Vega wrote in her song 'Language', 'I won't use words again; they don't mean what I meant.'[7]

Theories provide maps for problems whose meaning may be obscure. They help to anchor a therapist in the face of what initially makes no sense. They provide a scaffolding that can hold both therapist and client through difficult times.

I experienced training in several therapeutic approaches. Gestalt therapy helped me personally to reconnect with feelings in myself that I had disowned. It also enabled me to make others aware of and release hurt feelings they had been carrying for years. But my interventions had no guiding strategy or overall plan. When powerful emotions were released, I was often unsure where to go next.

CBT was ideal for someone like me who needed a more orderly way of engaging a person safely in therapy. It offered a more structured approach that linked childhood experiences, current life circumstances and behaviour.

CBT is one example of what are broadly described as 'brief' psychotherapies. These approaches work in a time-limited way and focus on strengthening a person's sense of Self. They aim to restore self-confidence and empower people to get on with their lives. But these therapies often fail to touch a person's fundamental sense of inadequacy, what the Hungarian psychoanalyst Michael Balint called 'a basic fault'. This refers to a feeling many of us share that something is not quite right inside us. Balint believed it most likely stems from some disruptive trauma in our earliest childhood. While brief forms of therapy may be very effective in getting people back on their feet, this underlying sense of being damaged may persist. Unconsciously, a person may continue to identify with the lack in themselves that they are trying to overcome.

Theories raise hypotheses about what may be going on inside or around a person. Perhaps this person's depression is a reflection of blocked grief, a deplorable self-image, or some loss which they deny upset them as much as it did. Perhaps another person's anxiety has little to do with what they are afraid may happen to them at some future point in their lives and everything to do with something that has already happened but has never been resolved. Perhaps an act of self-harm is how someone regulates their emotions when they become overwhelmed by them. Perhaps forgetfulness, checking out and dissociating are attempts to shut out memories they feel unready to face. Perhaps rage is a reaction to feeling completely disempowered in a toxic social situation.

The therapist and client form a trusting, collaborative alliance and become like two scientists or detectives who test a particular hypothesis or chase down possible reasons that may have disrupted this person's life.

But theories need to be absorbed and integrated so they become a silent backdrop to a therapist's work rather than flags they wave in therapy. When we take our theories too seriously, they can bias us in our work. The psychologist, Marilyn Charles, wrote:

> To some extent, we need to be willing to cast ourselves adrift from our theories to discover when, whether, and in what ways our theories apply. Otherwise, it becomes too easy merely to affirm what we already believe we know rather than learning anything from the actual experience.[8]

My strength as a therapist has always been a well-tuned intuition. Empathy always came easy to me. But it took me years to trust these qualities. As a novice, I discounted them as almost 'unprofessional' and worked hard to master specific therapeutic techniques and apply them diligently. Having specific interventions I could execute gave me, in my own mind, legitimacy as a therapist. But sometimes, my theories blinded me to what was right before me. An example that comes to mind is my work with a young girl called Susan.

Susan was fourteen and the daughter of a colleague. Susan's mother came to my office one day to discuss her daughter's intense fear of spiders. Her phobia was so bad that she spent two hours every night checking her bedroom for spiders before even considering sleeping. I had just completed my training in CBT and felt confident I could help her. I was sure that gradual desensitisation – the process of gradually exposing a person to increasingly fear-provoking situations until their fears subsided – was the key.

I saw her in my office and began by having her sit in the room with a plastic spider in a sealed container. She was terrified, but over time her anxiety eased, and she began to feel comfortable sitting in the room with my fake spider. Each week we raised the stakes. At some point, I invited her to bring her best friend to help her with being exposed to real spiders. Her friend's presence was both a support for Susan and a way to model for her another person being touched by a spider and nothing bad happening. I allowed a live spider to crawl over my wrist and onto her friend's wrist. After some time, I had the spider cross from her wrist (very quickly) to her friend's wrist. She gradually became comfortable with having a spider touch her skin through repeated exposure.

I had an endless supply of relatively large spiders at the time because St James's Hospital was a building site, with old units being torn down and new departments being erected. I never wanted to harm these spiders, so at the end of each session, I accompanied Susan as she released each spider in exactly the place where I'd found it. Taking care of the spiders had a curious impact on Susan. She began to see them as living beings in their own right who deserved the same care and respect that we all need.

I asked her mother to join us for her final session. After seven weeks, Susan showed her how she had become perfectly comfortable with two spiders crawling up each of her bare arms simultaneously. Everybody was impressed; I was thrilled.

At the session's close, I asked Susan to stay back a minute or two. I wanted some feedback and assumed it would be positive. I was wrong. Susan may have been afraid of spiders, but she wasn't afraid to speak her mind truthfully. She told me that she had been riddled with anxiety for the past year, but she had been able to project all her fears onto spiders. Now she knew it had never really been about spiders, but she had no idea how to handle her continuing anxiety. Her words came as a shock. I realised that I had completely missed what was going on in Susan's life. I felt both stupid and sad. I began to recall several off-hand remarks that both she and her mother had made and which I had chosen to ignore as I kept my eyes on the task we had set for ourselves. What was the threat in her life that she hadn't been able to articulate? I never found out, because I never saw her again.

Therapy is more an art than a science. There is no shortage of programmes that promise to steer the process neatly towards the desired destination of a depression-free, anxiety-free, robust self-image. In reality, it is never that straightforward. The experience can be slow and fraught with unintended misunderstandings on both sides.

The hurt that people bring to therapy usually gets played out in their relationship with the therapist. Indeed, a good therapist counts on this happening because it reveals the person's experience of relationships. Difficulty with trust, or a flare of anger in response to even the tiniest misunderstandings, can be a window to real-life experiences. Ruptures in the client–therapist relationship can serve as reality checks if we can handle the anger or disappointment they provoke without becoming defensive. Such ruptures create an opportunity to address the reality that people can let us down. Therapists make mistakes, and misunderstandings occur in every relationship, but in therapy, a person can address these ruptures rather than silently swallow their pain. One practice I have found very helpful as a therapist is asking a person at the close of a session for their feedback. I want to know what has been helpful, but more than that, I want to know if anything about the session made them uncomfortable. Positive feedback is reassuring, but negative feedback is gold because it opens an opportunity to discuss something we have no idea caused unintended distress.

Psychotherapy has become radically time-limited over the last decade or two. Brief, 'evidence-based' interventions have become the dominant form of therapy. The value of brief therapeutic models such as CBT are based on the finding that they improved a person's mood in highly controlled settings over 8–12 weeks. This was most often the case with people whose emotional distress was uncomplicated by social disadvantage, addiction, poverty or complex mental health issues. People's problems are usually a lot 'messier' in the real world. Brief interventions may help people to take back control, teach them important self-care skills and lift their morale. But they may fail to touch hidden layers of hurt. Many people need support on a long-term basis to enable them to come to terms with deeper wounds in their personal and social lives. They need someone in their lives who will 'have their back' over time until they can find in themselves the confidence they need to 'go it alone'. Today, having a consistent relationship over time with any kind of professional healthcare worker is perceived as a luxury we can't afford. But the need for this kind of consistent support is still there.

Psychotherapy is a very specialised skill. We hone our therapy skills in the field by working with real people in distress and being carefully supervised. Competent clinicians learn to hold their preferred theories lightly. Through reflecting in supervision on what happens – or doesn't happen – with clients, they learn from experience. They discover that each person who turns to them for help brings with them a unique set of challenges and learning opportunities.

Despite the differing theories underpinning them, at the heart of every therapeutic approach is an invitation to a person to connect with themselves and feel what is happening in their bodies and minds. Trauma makes it especially difficult to recognise our needs and feelings. Trauma makes us strangers to ourselves. It becomes possible to see what remains unresolved or unaddressed through awareness and acceptance of what is happening at any moment. Awareness is fundamental to being able to steady our emotions, to self-regulate. Difficulties in self-regulation are at the core of most severe mental health difficulties.

How do we help people to reconnect with themselves and become aware of what is happening to them? We usually need to first identify and examine their fears of exploring their inner experience. They may have been told to stay away from their inner lives because there is too much darkness there. Knowing when it's safe to move towards, rather than away, from that darkness requires skill. The delicacy required in therapy is to 'read' where someone is in their relationship with themselves and their readiness to explore painful issues.

Over the years, I have come to regard 'being present' as the central discipline of psychotherapy. Bion set every therapist the challenge 'to try to be as fully as possible in the moment, without regard to one's ideas about how or what one should or might be, without memory or desire.' Our presence is a mark of respect to the person speaking to us. It invites them to be present to themselves and attend more keenly to whatever is happening inside them.

I make the encounter as relaxed as possible in sessions. I keep my mind loose, so I don't focus on a specific problem prematurely. I have learned that the first issue a person presents with is rarely the problem; the real problem is usually held back until they have tested us and ensured we are not overly judgemental. Noticing how it feels to be in the room with a person is also a rich source of information that should be respected. My reactions to *this* person, here and now, may hold clues to what is happening either in them or to some dynamic unfolding between us.

I was fortunate to attend a weekend workshop the Scottish psychiatrist RD Laing gave at St James's Hospital in 1985. Someone in our small group asked him, 'What is psychotherapy?' In reply, he confessed that despite being asked that question a thousand times, he could never give an entirely satisfactory answer. Not that he didn't know the textbook definitions of psychotherapy, but that he regarded them all as falling short in terms of conveying what the experience felt like to both parties involved. The answer he gave that Saturday morning seemed to come to him in the moment. He replied, 'Somebody said somewhere, "Where two or three are gathered in my name, there I am among them". This captured what I believe is essential about therapy.'

I've reflected a lot on what he meant by quoting that particular piece of scripture. I think he was trying to convey something about the quality of presence that psychotherapy requires. For Laing, there was something profoundly personal about therapy. The somewhat technical language we use to describe the relationship in psychotherapy – 'therapeutic alliance', 'containment', 'corrective emotional experience' – doesn't quite reflect the magic that occurs when two people are present, aware and open to each other in a deeply respectful way. A therapist may hold the dignity of a person in distress when they cannot see it for themselves. Therapy provides a safe space for people to explore their insecurities and develop new skills to manage their lives. But what may be even more powerful are the creative insights that emerge within a therapy session that no one expects. Good therapy is reciprocal. The process changes both parties. Both learn from the experience.

I think that writers like Bion seek to remind us that, while language can give us a helpful map of a person's distress, it is never the territory. Psychotherapy requires the discipline of presence, openness and awareness. What emerges when we can be with someone in this way – and they, in turn, are present to their own experience – will almost always surprise us. Marylin Charles trained with Bion and now works as a psychoanalyst with people burdened by complex mental health challenges. Her first book on psychotherapy, *Learning from Experience,* is an excellent primer for anyone trying to deepen their understanding of psychotherapy. It closes with the following quote:

> So, I would tell you not to worry too much about the language or the theory or what you think you're

supposed to be doing. Gird yourself sufficiently that you can have a good-enough story going to tolerate the discomfort as you build a better one, one that more clearly fits the facts of yourself and your patients as you go about this arduous but very rewarding business of finding your way through.[9]

9

PERSONAL THERAPY

As long as the pain borne of the past is denied, there
will be someone paying the price in terms of sanity.[1]

ALICE MILLER

Psychotherapy becomes important when our friendships, close relationships and the natural resources we rely on to keep us grounded – our connection with nature, our pets, our favourite sport, our love of reading or music – fail to help us resolve some particular issue in our lives. Psychotherapy can help us write a new story of who we are. In the words of Wilfred Bion, it can 'suddenly introduce order where the appearance of disorder has reigned.'[2] For my personal therapy, I turned to psychoanalysis.

Psychoanalysis is a form of psychotherapy that believes our mood and our behaviour are influenced by memories, traumas, unresolved conflicts and needs that we are unaware of. These powerful forces in the mind reside in the unconscious. A psychoanalyst is a therapist skilled in creating the conditions within which the unconscious can reveal itself. By making the unconscious conscious, a person achieves important insights into their feelings about themselves and how they relate to others. They can identify and address what has been hidden and inaccessible. The aim of psychoanalysis is greater freedom to choose how we want to live, rather than be pushed around by forces we don't understand.

Psychoanalysis takes time. It only works when there is deep trust between the patient and the analyst. I knew how big a commitment this was and also what a privilege it was to be able to work on one's issues in such a slow, careful way. I wanted to be sure the therapist I picked was someone I felt at ease with, at the very least.

I arranged a single exploratory session with three eminent psychoanalysts. The first two therapists I visited asked me many questions and finished with a summary of what they regarded as my core 'issues'. Their summations didn't feel quite right. They felt premature. The third person I visited was someone with a much lower profile than the first two. I knew hardly anything about her. But I spent most of our introductory session in tears. When it was over, we agreed on a follow-up appointment. I left knowing that this was the person for me. My unconscious had felt safe with her. My tears were evidence of how secure I felt in her presence. Her silence and unintrusive presence felt immensely respectful.

As a card-carrying cognitive-behavioural therapist – indeed, the director at that point of a postgraduate MSc in Cognitive Psychotherapy at Trinity College, Dublin – this was not something I imagined I would ever do. Over the course of my career, it had become fashionable for enlightened psychologists to parody psychoanalysis and dismiss it as a middle-class indulgence with no evidence base. And yet I found myself, by choice, lying on a couch, with my therapist sitting behind me, freely associating about my life, and experiencing intense pain and emotion that I'd been carrying all my life.

I had several reasons for choosing analysis. I had been pushed around since childhood by feelings of sadness and shame that made no sense to me. I believed something was fundamentally broken in me. Talking about myself at different periods with counsellors and therapists hadn't gotten me to the heart of why I felt so bad. I needed to go deeper.

I was also a course director with many students who were counting on me to enable them to become competent therapists. I was teaching and supervising them weekly. Supervision carries with it serious responsibilities. I could unwittingly pass on my prejudices and blind spots to them. I needed to know myself better so this wouldn't happen.

Analysis with Ann, a Kleinian psychoanalyst, took me into places I never anticipated I would go. We slowly explored deeper into my early childhood. I remembered and relived painful episodes I'd buried long ago and reopened many old wounds. It taught me to sit with my pain, to feel what I felt and experience what happened when I did. Therapy also exposed my dark side. I was prone to jealousy. I was angry in a way that didn't fit my 'nice guy' image. I had a hard time trusting people. I didn't trust myself or what I felt in my body. I didn't trust my own voice – I wasn't even sure that I had one. I mimicked the views and opinions of people and writers I admired. I couldn't make decisions. Most of all, I hated my inability to find peace. My mother-in-law had always said I was a 'tortured soul'. She was right.

I had 'breakthrough' moments in the course of my sessions with Ann. On one such occasion, she invited me to explore my feelings about my brother Jim. What emerged were mixed feelings of love and grief, envy and jealousy. I loved him as a brother, but he was also the apple of my mother's eye, a rival for the affections of a woman I had entirely to myself until he arrived. As a blond, curly-haired boy, he'd won the hearts of uncles and aunts who adored him. My therapist suggested that while I'd loved him, it was possible that I also had moments of wishing he wasn't there. 'And then', she added, 'the day came when he wasn't.' I had struggled with feelings of rivalry for my entire adult life. Acknowledging that I had once been jealous of the little brother I tragically lost allowed me to 'let go' of some of that burden.

Therapy gave me the experience of being with someone who gave me the right amount of space – not so much that I felt abandoned, not so little that it was filled with someone else's ideas – to gradually find and speak in my own voice. I attended for six years because it took that long for me to confront and integrate elements of my inner world and to grow up. Even then, she and I agreed I wasn't ready to terminate. We stopped only because she left Ireland to take a sabbatical abroad. I was still raw then and continued to be for several years afterwards.

Ann was eager for me to transfer to someone else, but that felt like a bridge too far. One of the reasons it is so important to put careful boundaries around therapy relationships is that they can become so intimate. Ann was the most professional therapist I've ever met; she was very private and generally said very little. She did nothing to encourage emotional dependency. Our final session ended like any other, with a gracious goodbye. She had arranged for a colleague of hers to continue with me. But I had developed an intense bond of trust with her. When we finished, I needed time to grieve her loss. I couldn't start over with someone else.

Through psychoanalysis, I learned how powerfully my earliest experiences had shaped my life. The reach of our unresolved wounds should never be underestimated. We don't forget, overcome or erase difficulties in our past; instead, we face them. We feel them, or we are forever ruled by them. We invite our traumas in from the cold and make them part of our identity. We befriend them so that they no longer wander like outlaws in the hinterland of our unconscious, erupting occasionally and raising havoc. We accept ourselves. But first, we need to face ourselves and know ourselves.

I understand now that the worst part of my early hospitalisations and separations was my struggle to manage the emotional chaos I felt afterwards. I was left to my own devices.

The best coping skills I could come up with were those of a child: withdrawal and self-soothing. I experienced my various separations as a form of abandonment that felt irreversible. But that needn't have been so. Their impact would have been very different if someone, ideally my parents, could have recognised my distress and actively helped me to cope. Times of disruption and pain do not have to shut us down. We are at our most vulnerable when our hearts are broken open, but those moments are also when we are most poised to grow. We discover what really matters and how much we need each other.

In so far as I've been able to face and come to terms with events in my past, I've been able to make choices about how I want to live in the present. My resistance to dealing with difficulty has formed some kind of alliance with the resilience in me that never gave up on my search for Self. As this self has grown stronger – which largely has meant being more honest and accepting of my vulnerabilities – I have made different choices in how I wanted to live and become much more at ease in my own skin.

What I remember most from my sessions with Ann was how cold I felt when I left her office. Some days, I walked out into beautiful summer days and shivered all the way home like someone who had forgotten to bring a coat on a frosty mid-winter day. I was chilled to the core, but I also had greater confidence to be more open and honest in my relationship with myself and others.

Those years were some of the hardest in my life. But it was also, ironically, during those years that I left St James's and established the youth mental health service Headstrong, later to be renamed Jigsaw. Some years later, Ursula and I both committed to a course of marital therapy which took several years. We gradually found a way of being married that works for us both.

Some issues are tougher than others to resolve. Therapy rarely offers quick fixes for the problems that originally motivated us to seek help, but it does allow us to gradually understand what is happening and why we are behaving the way we are. Both Ursula and I had as good an experience of therapy as one could hope for. I am much clearer now than I was then about the responsibilities that come with important and intimate relationships. Therapy points us in a general direction of where solutions may lie, but it does not promise us easy answers.

DIGNITY IN MADNESS

Working with an individual with problems – rather than problematising him – is an ongoing challenge in an age in which distress and disorder are thought of as aberrant phenomena to be eradicated by whatever means we have at hand.[1]

MARILYN CHARLES

n the week before Christmas 2000, a man in his late thirties entered my office. His name was David. He sat slumped in the chair, looking miserable. He said he felt like he was drowning in despair.

David was prone to radical mood swings. For some years, his life had alternated between times when he felt euphoric and full of energy and periods when he felt utterly forlorn and hopeless. Sitting in my office that day, he seemed completely dejected. 'I have two options,' he said, 'I either come back into hospital or take the jar of medication I've been hoarding beside my bed to end this pain.'

Neither option sounded good to me. David had already spent most of that year in the hospital and had been a familiar face in our service for the previous 10 years. It was hard to believe that another admission would make any real difference in his life. His plan B looked even less attractive.

We sat together in the pall of his gloom. We talked about what triggered this downturn in his life and he described a series of little things that had gotten to him. 'My thoughts and feelings are pushing me around, and I'm pissed off with it all.' He knew that he was overreacting to these thoughts, but he couldn't get them out of his head. He was exhausted by his inner turmoil. Heavy doses of medication were making very little difference. He needed some practical ways to calm himself and take back control over his life. And then an idea struck me.

I first read about mindfulness in *Full Catastrophe Living* by Jon Kabat-Zinn in 1994. There was something different in how Jon described dealing with physical pain in a medical setting, I didn't completely understand his approach at the time, but I was intrigued by his writing. I also couldn't see how his approach could be helpful to people with complex and persistent mental health problems. So the book had sat undisturbed for six years on my bookshelf in St James's Hospital.

Taking *Full Catastrophe Living* down from its shelf – and dusting it off – I opened it and scanned its contents for something I remembered that Jon Kabat-Zinn had written. David needed a radically different way to think about himself and his problems. I found the page and read aloud the section I'd marked six years earlier:

> When we glimpse our completeness in the stillness of any moment, when we directly experience ourselves during the body scan or sitting, or while practising yoga, as a whole at that moment and also as part of a larger whole, a new and profound coming to terms with our problems and our suffering begins to take place. We begin to see both ourselves and our problems differently, namely from the perspective of wholeness. This transformation of view creates an entirely different context within which we can see and work with our problems, however serious they might be. It is a perceptual shift away from fragmentation and isolation toward wholeness and connectedness. With this change of perspective comes a shift from feeling out of control and beyond help (helpless and pessimistic) to a sense of the possible, a sense of acceptance and inner peace and control. Healing always involves an emotional and attitudinal transformation.[2]

When I first read this passage, I was struck by its hope. We prided ourselves in the hospital on being able to dissect and label what was wrong with people, and we usually made rather pessimistic predictions regarding their likelihood of recovery. But Kabat-Zinn took as his starting point the fundamental truth that we are whole, complete and connected, and that our problems, however serious they might be, are workable.

David liked the sound of this. I photocopied the full chapter and a few simple exercises he could practice at home. I was never comfortable asking someone to do something that I hadn't yet fully mastered, but we both felt these exercises were worth a try.

We returned to the bottle of pills he'd been collecting beside his bed. He wasn't willing to ditch them but agreed to lock them away. He would also talk to his community nurse, with whom he had a very open, trusting relationship. He would ask him to stop by his home over the holiday to check his progress. I also promised to check in with him.

When David returned to my office in the new year, he seemed brighter. He was standing straighter and there was a smile on his face. He reported feeling better and attributed his improvement to the practical comfort he found in the material I'd photocopied from *Full Catastrophe Living*. He was ready for the next instalment.

This pattern of photocopying selected texts and exercises continued for several weeks until one day David sat opposite me with a very serious expression on his face. He looked me straight in the eye and said, 'This stuff is really important. You need to read it.' I replied that I had read it some years ago, but David wasn't impressed. 'This is different to anything we've ever talked about. You need to really know about it,' he repeated.

A few months later, I attended an annual psychotherapy conference in the UK where a flier caught my eye. It was for an eight-day Mindfulness-Based Stress Reduction training course given by Jon Kabat-Zinn and another mindfulness expert, Saki Santorelli, at the University of Bangor in North Wales. Destiny was knocking on my door. I signed up and my career as a clinical psychologist took a whole new direction.

The Department of Psychiatry, Trinity College, in St James's Hospital Dublin, hosted a community-based mental health service for Dublin's city centre and several of its adjoining neighbourhoods. It was a 50-bed hospital, with a locked 25-bed ward upstairs and a more open-day hospital downstairs. The latter had an occupational therapy department, group therapy rooms and an impressive woodwork suite.

Having completed the MBSR training with Jon Kabat-Zinn, I enrolled in a teacher's course in Mindfulness-Based Cognitive Therapy (MBCT). Part of the programme required me to run an eight-week mindfulness group under supervision. In the weeks leading up to our start date, I'd explained mindfulness to the hospital staff and invited referrals to this 'pilot' programme. I suspect they had no idea what I was talking about – in 2002, mindfulness was a word that had to be followed every time with a lengthy explanation. It wasn't the household name that it is today. Most of my colleagues interpreted what I planned to do as a form of enhanced 'relaxation training', and felt that this certainly couldn't do anyone any harm.

One man approached me on his own initiative and asked to be included in the group. I didn't know him well at the time, but I had often noticed him around the hospital. Simon had been a user of our in-patient and community services for as long as I could remember. His favourite perch was a windowsill along the entrance corridor to the hospital, where he sat for long stretches. I'd passed him so often that I'd stopped noticing him. I wonder how many other people I stopped noticing over the years because their admissions had become so routine that their presence didn't surprise me.

Simon had first been admitted to a psychiatric hospital at age 14 and had been admitted a further 18 times. He had accumulated almost as many diagnoses, each one sounding more ominous than the one before. It can be hard, at first, to see beyond such labels; a person can become easily lost behind the ominous-sounding language of psychopathology. I saw a large man in his thirties with a warm smile.

Simon was keen to join the mindfulness group, but I wasn't sure it was what he needed. He spoke with his team about it the next day. I suspect they shared my hesitation but believed it couldn't hurt. The consensus among staff was that his recovery had gone as far as it could. There was no great expectation that he could progress much further. The goal of his treatment was to reduce his relapse rate as far as possible.

So Simon became a member of that group, along with 11 other long-term service users, most of whom were well-known to him. This included David, who was his close friend and who had encouraged him to give it a chance. After all, he had practised mindfulness before any of us, and he had great faith in it.

The 12 group members could have written a textbook on severe and enduring mental health difficulties between them. They had weathered repeated psychotic breakdowns, depression, anxiety and trauma. They looked apprehensive as we gathered for the opening session. No one knew what we had let ourselves in for. The unspoken question on all our minds was, 'Could mindfulness make any difference to deep-seated emotional problems?'

The eight-week MBCT course took us 10 weeks to complete. There was a lot of material to get through, and I didn't want to rush things. Regarding the suggested 'homework' between sessions, we agreed on what was realistic rather than recommended in the manual. For example, David suggested we commit to a daily three-minute meditation practice, to begin with. The important thing was that we practised whatever we committed to every day.

As the course progressed, the time people spent completing the daily practice activities (movement exercises, sitting practice, reading and recording thoughts and feelings) naturally increased. When the course ended, most of the group spent 20 minutes practising mindfulness daily.

I ran every type of group therapy programme over the 30 years I served in James's hospital. Running the MBCT group felt different to all the rest. I was the leader, but we were all equal. For the group to work, we had to be honest with each other about our experience of learning to meditate. We all had our 'bad' weeks when practice didn't happen or didn't go well. We encouraged each small step in our collective progress.

Mindfulness gave us a new way of relating to ourselves. Instead of trying to 'fix' our problems, we learned to give them room to breathe. And when we felt uncomfortable or got carried away by thoughts, we returned our attention to breathing and gave our minds time to settle. Sometimes we imagined our negative thoughts as buses passing in front of our minds. They were just thoughts, not truths. We could recognise them and acknowledge them, but we didn't have to climb on board. Our mantra became, 'Feel what you feel, but let go of the story'.

Many people in the group described how they'd been made to feel very cautious about their inner lives. They had heard that self-examination could undo whatever defences they had put in place to repress distressing memories and unresolved conflict. For most of my career as a staff psychologist, people vulnerable to psychosis were considered off-limits when it came to psychotherapy. People prone to psychosis were known to be incredibly sensitive. They were perceived as having difficulty coping with emotionally loaded situations. Families where there was an intense emotional atmosphere tended to result in a higher number of relapses for people diagnosed with schizophrenia than families which were mostly calm. Individual therapy was discouraged because of the risk it could provoke painful memories and emotional distress. This could inadvertently cause relapse.

But here we were together, learning the art of moving towards, rather than away from, distress. We were miners bringing the lamp of awareness into places previously identified as no-go territory.

This was all more radical than I initially realised, but the MBCT programme is designed very thoughtfully to avoid people becoming overwhelmed. The first four sessions of the programme gave exclusive attention to breathing, settling the body and connecting with our bodies through movement and walking. We were halfway through the course before inviting people to become aware of their emotions.

Mindfulness also taught people to be compassionate with their vulnerabilities rather than critical, to be patient rather than pester themselves for their failings. The group gradually named and shared losses and disappointments in their lives. They spoke of their dreams and their regrets with one another. They also learned to notice what made them happy and to plan for times when they would do something enjoyable. The gentleness in how they engaged with their emotions, the structure of each group meeting and the quiet room where we convened all contributed to creating a 'holding' space where participants felt safe and secure.

Mindfulness helped this group to be less afraid of themselves and taught them how to steady themselves in stressful situations. After years of hearing that their inner lives could not be trusted, they found a safe way to befriend parts of themselves from which they had become alienated. Trust came slowly through brief moments where they acknowledged and allowed themselves to feel what they felt and not push it away.

Some people in the group needed a second round of sessions to achieve trust in their inner lives. They needed more time to befriend themselves and learn how to care for themselves. David and Simon were two people who appreciated a chance to consolidate their mindfulness by repeating the course.

I'd worked in psychiatric hospitals for 25 years before I incorporated mindfulness into my work. Throughout that time, people in acute emotional distress were referred to me for therapy. Relieving their pain was considered the priority. What mental health professionals often failed to appreciate, however, was that rage and grief were as inevitable when healing from psychological trauma as pain and discomfort are when recovering from a physical injury. Ironically, psychiatric hospitals were not places where you were 'allowed' to be upset. The first sign of distress, anger or sadness generally triggered the appearance of your team, armed with every medical resource available to take away your pain.

Our mindfulness groups gave people a safe way to acknowledge their feelings without being overwhelmed by them. It didn't offer explanations or quick fixes to anyone who became upset. Instead, it showed people how to be with distressing emotions, respect them, and listen to what those feelings were trying to communicate.

On day seven of every MBCT course, the class gathered for a full day to consolidate the different mindfulness skills to which they had been introduced. For our group, I rented a meditation centre outside Dublin surrounded by fields and overlooking the sea. There were spaces to meet, eat and walk silently during the day.

After lunch, I joined Simon on the outside porch and asked him how he was doing. I'd been unsure whether he was benefitting from the classes, although he seemed to enjoy them. I asked him directly how helpful he found them.

Simon was taken aback by my question. He detailed a number of changes that had happened since joining the course: his medication had been halved; he'd moved into independent, supported accommodation; he was volunteering in a local club; and he had registered with the Open University to study specific subjects that would allow him, aged 34, to complete his unfinished secondary school education. Then he told me the following story.

He had recently taken a train from Dublin's city centre to visit a friend in Bray. Sitting in one of the carriages as the train moved from one station to the next, he started worrying about all he had to do in the days ahead. He became absorbed in his thoughts and less aware of the people around him. He described a moment where some sound, perhaps the screech of wheels on tracks, startled him. Looking up, gripped by anxiety, he saw blue rays of light streaming from the eyes of some of his fellow passengers.

His first instinct was to get away as fast as he could. He was agitated and frightened, but in that same moment, he recognised what was happening. And he remembered something he'd learned in our mindfulness classes. He planted his feet on the floor, lowered his gaze, and focused on breathing. He allowed the simple rhythm of his breathing to steady him gradually. After a few minutes, he soothingly spoke to himself. 'You're over-stressed; you're trying to do too much, and you keep pushing yourself to do more. You need to stop, slow down and give your body a chance to catch up.'

He sat quietly for a few minutes, head down, and let the emotional storm inside him settle. His breathing slowed, and he felt himself calming down. In his own time, he opened his eyes and looked up. The carriage was still full of people, but there were no blue lights.

As we spoke about this experience, Simon emphasised that this was a small miracle. 'Before I learned to recognise and take care of my stress,' he said, 'that story would have had a very different ending. I would have reacted to seeing lights by standing up and changing carriages at the next station. And in that carriage, everyone's eyes would have had blue light streaming. So, I would have jumped off the train at the next stop and run home because I couldn't trust any public transport. I'd have locked myself in my room and climbed under the covers, and my fears would have taken hold of me. After a few days, the community nurse would have been called, and I'd have been admitted to the hospital, where I would stay for up to nine months.'

Simon's first hospital admission at age 14 had been to an adult in-patient ward in St Ita's Hospital, Portrane. Despite receiving what he described as excellent care there, there were many repeat hospital admissions over the years. Now he had begun to wonder why his treatment had never included a way to cope with stress and anxiety. Why had no one helped him make sense of his extreme reactions, hallucinations and paranoia? Why had no one ever tried to teach him to manage his stress?

I knew the answer to this. Usually, in the case of someone like Simon, the question, 'Why not refer them for a course of therapy to explore what triggers their distress and give them skills to manage it?' is met with the response, 'This person is too sick to benefit from therapy' or 'Their past is not the problem here, it's their brain chemistry.'

The only way to be sure that mindfulness had helped Simon, rather than the various psychotropic medications he took daily, would have been to discontinue all of them and see how he fared. This would of course have been unethical, but in the case of Simon, it happened. He had to discontinue his medications because he was diagnosed with pancreatic cancer two years later.

When I heard the news of his diagnosis, it had been a while since I'd been with Simon. I went to the hospital and found him lying in a bed, alone in a single room in the cancer ward. I barely recognised him. He had lost several stone in weight, but what surprised me most was how cheerful he was. He joked that he'd been attending 'shrinks' for years, but all they had done was 'expand' him. Then he looked at me and asked me how things were going for me. That wasn't an easy subject to talk about. I was in a hard place. I was living alone away from my family and I seemed unable to resolve several painful issues in my personal life. My problems seemed minor compared to Simon's, and I didn't want to add to his concerns. But from the serious look on his face, I felt he deserved nothing less than an honest answer.

So, I spoke to him about my life. And the tears came. Much more powerfully than I had expected or wanted. He listened. His warmth was a poultice to my pain. When I regained my composure, he lay in the bed looking at me with understanding. He didn't press me to say any more than I wanted.

All of Simon's medications had been discontinued, but he still received frequent visits from his community nurse, Michael O'Driscoll. Their relationship was special and had sustained Simon through many dark periods of his life. His face broke into a smile when I asked him how he felt.

Mindfulness was keeping him together, he said. His mood was steady. He wasn't so frightened by his paranoid thoughts anymore. He accepted that they came and went and, if necessary, he checked them out. If he felt people were talking about him or he sensed some hidden derogatory message in what they were saying, he asked them directly what they meant. He could see now that his paranoia was a projection of his inner insecurities out into the world. He worked hard to understand his fears, treating them with patience and kindness while not allowing them to take over. His psychosis had become his imagination.

It undoubtedly helped that Simon now had a 'proper', socially recognised illness with a relatable social identity. Suddenly he was no longer the 'crazy man in the corner'; he was a cancer patient, someone with whom we could all empathise. As upsetting as his illness was, it was not something to be feared.

Without his medications, his family and medical team feared the worst for Simon. But to their surprise, he was fine. He said he felt better without them and credited his mindfulness practice for this. He even steered his family towards various mindfulness courses.

Simon was discharged two months later. His cancer wasn't getting better, but it seemed to have plateaued. He was in no pain, and his general mood was very good, so I asked him if he'd like to help me with a new group I was about to run. I'd been asked to run a pilot MBCT group in an addiction centre in one of Dublin's toughest inner-city neighbourhoods. I invited both Simon and David to co-lead this group with me.

Our group comprised 14 men and women, most of them HIV positive, all of them with severe, life-threatening addictions. They had reached a point where relapse was a luxury they couldn't afford. For these men and women, mindfulness wasn't some new gimmick. It offered hope that they could avoid a relapse that would likely kill them.

We followed the same format, pretty much, that we'd followed in James's. I also asked a yoga instructor friend, Orla Punch, to help with the movement aspect of mindfulness training, and that component of the course was a major hit. Faye Scanlan, a young, recently-qualified psychologist, was the fifth member of the team with responsibility for gathering data and evaluating the course. After each session, we made a point of sitting down and debriefing. What worked, what hadn't worked, what had we learned?

Simon and David played a key role in the group by sharing what had been helpful to each of them in learning to meditate and the difference it had made to their mental health. But on week six, Simon spoke personally about his life before mindfulness and the medical challenges he was now facing.

He started by explaining what had drawn him to mindfulness. After 20 years of severe psychotic episodes and annual hospital admissions, it had given him the skills he needed to steady himself when he became distressed and paranoid. His gentleness, combined with a very infectious sense of humour, made his recovery sound a lot easier than it had been. But this group picked up on how tough it had been.

And then Simon delivered his 'punch line': 'It's taken me years to sort out my life, and now I feel I'm doing very well. But the funny thing is that as soon as I got over my mental problems, I developed a slight physical problem that I will probably not shake off. A year ago, I was diagnosed with pancreatic cancer.'

He smiled when he said this, perhaps to lessen the blow of his words. But no one else was smiling. There wasn't a dry eye in the room. These were hardened souls, but even the hardest among them cried openly. Their respect for Simon had grown over the course, and they were genuinely sorry for what lay ahead of him.

But Simon didn't want his story to have a tragic ending. He said that he felt happier now than he ever had in his life. He was at peace in his mind and wasn't in any pain. All he asked of life was that he could have until after Christmas that year. He had a 'bucket list' to complete. This included a road trip with his brother to visit family in the Netherlands and the UK.

At 37 years old, Simon looked like the happy and fresh-faced young boy he'd never had the chance to be. He'd finally become himself; nothing more but nothing less. And he taught me the value of meditation more than any teacher I've ever had.

Simon died peacefully on 27 December 2007, with all the items on his bucket list ticked off. David and I spent time with him briefly in the hospital the day before he died. His family, whom he loved, accompanied him in his final hours. At the funeral, they mentioned how mindfulness had been so important to him and joked about how he'd insisted they also had to learn to practise it.

I remembered the question I'd asked him, sitting on that porch four years earlier: Was mindfulness helping him? He had answered it powerfully with his life and his death.

On that occasion, he also told me that he had watched me as I passed him by on his windowsill for years. He could read my mood by the way I walked, the angle of my head and the expression on my face. He would feel concerned when he noticed I was stressed and tired, while I, the 'professional', didn't even notice him there, lost somewhere inside my head.

Simon had no further breakdowns or hospital admissions before his death. His experience of recovery – after 20 years of treatment for major psychotic breakdowns – raises the question of whether the despair we generate around people diagnosed with psychosis reflects the poverty of our imagination rather than the nature of this form of human suffering.

Over the years, as our relationship deepened, I had learned more about Simon's past. He was abused as a boy and had felt too shocked, ashamed and powerless to tell anyone. His growing isolation and guilt in his early teens eventually took their toll, eventually leading to that first hospital admission at age 14. His hospitalisation temporarily stopped the abuse, but after being discharged, it started up again. Simon carried this secret for years, partly to protect his family and because he believed it was his problem. His paranoia was perhaps a manifestation of the predator over which he had no control, a tormentor that could appear at any moment to punish him. Before he became physically unwell, Simon had discussed what had happened with his family. He also confronted his abuser in person.

In her book *Strangers to Ourselves,* the author Rachel Aviv poses fundamental questions about how we understand ourselves in periods of crisis and distress:

> Psychiatrists know remarkably little about why some people with mental illnesses recover and others with the same diagnosis go on to have an illness 'career'. Answering the question, I think, requires paying more attention to the distance between the psychiatric models that explain illness and the stories through which people find meaning. These stories alter people's lives and bear heavily on a person's sense of self – and the desire to be treated at all.[3]

What I have learned from working with people like Simon and David is that our predictions as to what is possible for them in terms of being well, being happy and creating a meaningful life for themselves are incredibly pessimistic. We conclude discharge summaries with some prognosis as to the likelihood of their recovery that reflects our lack of vision for them. For many people, hearing the term 'schizophrenia' is terrifying because it sounds so hopeless. I wanted to tell Simon's story because, for me, it shows that we don't always factor a person's strengths and talents into a recovery plan. We need to allow people to surprise us and prove us wrong – despite our imagined expertise in mental health. We do a person a grave injustice when we shut down possibilities for him or her achieving a greater depth of understanding for their vulnerabilities and the confidence and skill to manage them.

THOUGHTS ON PSYCHOSIS

There is a pain – so utter –
It swallows substance up –
Then covers the Abyss with Trance –
So Memory can step
Around – across – upon it –[1]

EMILY DICKINSON

An elegant lady in her late fifties seals the doors and windows of her flat to prevent toxic gas from leaking in. She believes that everyone in the apartment complex has joined forces and is planning to poison her. She can feel this in her bones. A bright university graduate feels terrified as he flees from every white van he sees in his neighbourhood. He is convinced the IRA are tailing him with the intent to kill him.

People can become psychotic when they are so overwhelmed by anxiety that they withdraw from reality. The capacity to think logically fractures into shards of images and thoughts that chase each other around their agitated minds. In response to a world that has suddenly become a major threat, they act in a way they believe can keep them safe. They may cling desperately to explanations for their being threatened, but their reasoning and defensive behaviours make no obvious sense. They can become isolated inside their torment, beyond the reach of even their most trusted friend.

The intensity of emotion they experience is unnerving to witness. But when the agitation passes, which it can do surprisingly quickly, what follows may be even more disconcerting. Their distress and agitation may give way to apathy and emptiness.

Their explanations of what is happening to them – 'people are trying to kill me', 'I have special powers that threaten other people' – sound incredible to family and friends, who regard them as delusions. Unable to relate to a loved one's bizarre take on reality, family and friends conclude that they've 'lost it'. But, despite their implausibility, delusions often give someone in psychological freefall some temporary stability.

Many life circumstances can lead to a psychotic break with reality. If a person remains vulnerable to experiencing repeated episodes of psychosis, they are often viewed as having a condition called schizophrenia. How exactly one person has an experience of psychosis and recovers, while someone else remains vulnerable to repeated episodes is not clear.

A young woman I worked with in James's described to me how she learned to take refuge from distress as a teenager by retreating into a world of beautiful hallucinations. This became her way of coping with agitation and restlessness. Initially, her withdrawal into fantasy gave her relief, but over time her sanctuary became a prison. Her hallucinations changed to something dark and hostile. She became a hostage to terrifying voices and visions that felt completely real. She was eventually admitted to hospital and diagnosed as having paranoid schizophrenia.

In his book *What is Madness?* psychoanalyst and writer Damien Leader describes this experience:

> The person may feel as if they are being duped, hypnotised, invaded, manipulated and deprived of their will ... the schizophrenic may feel subject to some outside power that controls them and can drop them at any time. They are in the position of an object, used by a powerful Other, perhaps with the idea of being their passive plaything.[2]

James Joyce's daughter Lucia fell hopelessly in love with Samuel Beckett when she was 20 and he was 21. However, he ended their relationship, possibly triggering an early psychotic breakdown for Lucia. Her behaviour became increasingly incomprehensible to her father, which prompted Joyce to arrange an appointment with the psychoanalyst Carl Jung. After meeting with each of them, Jung believed that Joyce and his daughter both had schizophrenia. He believed that Joyce's gift for language and writing saved him as it allowed him to communicate his experience, to use words to reconcile what for the rest of us may seem an unnameable chaos. Jung told Richard Ellmann, Joyce's biographer, that Lucia and James were 'like two people going to the bottom of a river, one falling and the other diving'.[3] Lucia died in 1982 after years of psychiatric institutionalisation. One of her very few visitors was Beckett.

Language, for all its many limitations, expresses our experience, shapes our reality and enables us to turn our conflicts into conversations. But where do we begin to convey such an experience in language? If we were as gifted as Beckett or Joyce, we might create a new language to express what was happening, even if it didn't conform to ordinary norms of speaking. And this is exactly what many people experiencing acute psychosis try to do. Because existing language falls so far short of the nightmare they find themselves in, they invent new ways of describing things that more closely express their feelings. But this new language locks them into another reality, making them feel isolated.

Psychosis is not a uniform phenomenon; it affects different people differently. A century of research has asked, 'What causes psychosis'? The answers have included genetic defects, chemical imbalances, poor parenting, depressed mothers, absent fathers, social deprivation, communication problems and trauma. Psychiatry has devoted much time over the past four decades to refining the diagnostic criteria for schizophrenia and antipsychotic medications. Today, it views the spectrum of psychotic disorders as genetically based and a manifestation of some neurological malfunction. No consistent objective evidence for either of these hypotheses has been identified. The truth is that we still don't know.

Advocates of the 'neurological malfunction' hypothesis like to compare slides of 'normal' brains with those diagnosed with schizophrenia. Their CT scans show differences, which is taken as definitive evidence that neurological abnormalities cause conditions such as schizophrenia. This may be a faulty conclusion because it ignores the fact that the human brain is designed to interact and survive in whatever kind of environment a person finds themselves in. Its nature is to respond and develop in line with what is happening in them and around them. Neuroplasticity has shown us how responsive the brain is to human experiences at every stage of our lives. Brain changes may be associated with mental and emotional pain, but that doesn't mean they explain them. The more fundamental question we need to ask is, 'What happened to this person in their lives to leave their brain the way it is?' Maybe that brain has been traumatised.

Psychological and social research has identified marginalisation, social isolation, and failure to mourn as key contributors to psychosis. There is a growing body of evidence that psychosis is trauma-driven. Psychologists and psychiatrists, including John Read, Ian Kelleher and Max Birchwood, uncovered different kinds of traumas in the lives of people with severe psychosis. Mostly, they were characterised by repeated aggressive or abusive actions in interpersonal situations, marked by power imbalances.[4] The experience of being bullied as a child was a consistent finding across these investigations.[5] Research in Ireland has shown that bullying is linked with a higher risk of psychotic illness in later life.[6]

Over time, the creators of the Diagnostic and Statistical Manual of Mental Disorders (also known as the DSM, and now in its fifth edition) have changed the criteria for diagnosis. What was called schizophrenia at one time might not be called schizophrenia at another. Current thinking requires that a person have hallucinations, delusions or disorganised speech that persists for at least a month and evidence of psychological or social deterioration for at least six months. Hearing voices has often been misdiagnosed as psychotic, but the evidence is that hearing voices is not enough to say someone has psychosis. About 15 per cent of people who feel anxious or depressed hear voices, and in times of great danger, people may hear voices that direct them towards a certain course of action.

Sometimes the hurts people experienced in the past come back to haunt them in curious ways. They may arise as thoughts that seem to come at them out of nowhere. They may include: 'It was my fault', 'I am so stupid', 'I made him do it', 'I'm filthy', and so on. A person may experience these thoughts as their own or as a voice spoken by someone else. The sudden eruption of these thoughts can be terrifying because they can appear when least expected and perhaps for no obvious reason. These thoughts may be like fragments of unintegrated memories seeking to find a home in our conscious lives.

Whatever combination of factors contributes to triggering schizophrenia, it has long been regarded as a psychic death sentence, which makes it a very hard diagnosis to hear for individuals and their families. It is mostly spoken about as a lifelong 'illness'. The advice is to stay close to one's psychiatric team, take strong medication which will likely cause significant side effects for the rest of one's life and maybe find some minimally stressful occupation. Family expectations for that person plummet and can become self-fulfilling.

Elyn Saks is a professor of law, psychology and psychiatry at the University of Southern California. In her memoir, *The Centre Cannot Hold: My Journey through Madness,* she writes that when she was diagnosed with schizophrenia, she felt as if she were 'being told that whatever had gone wrong inside my head was permanent and unfixable. Repeatedly, I ran up against words like 'debilitating', 'baffling', 'chronic', catastrophic', 'devastating' and 'loss'. For the rest of my life. *The rest of my life.*'[7]

Medications do seem to benefit people in the grip of psychosis. They take the edge off their distress, help them sleep and enable them to talk more easily about what is happening. Best practice is to start people on low doses and explain any possible side effects to the person and their family. A good physician also offers space for someone to talk about what they are going through.

Although beneficial and life-saving for many, psychotropic medications tend to be over-prescribed, leaving many individuals worse off.[8] At one time, progressive brain changes in people diagnosed with schizophrenia were interpreted as the cause of their schizophrenia, but later research concluded that these brain changes were more likely a side-effect of the antipsychotic medications these people received.[9]

Two Canadian psychiatrists, Guy Chouinard and Barry Jones, discovered that antipsychotic medications could induce a biological vulnerability to schizophrenia.[10] They describe how antipsychotics cause an increase in dopamine which, at some point, can become abnormal. When medications are discontinued, normal brain activity is disrupted, worsening symptoms. The brain seems to compensate by accelerating dopamine production. A person experiencing these effects can feel like they've lost a critical support system and become acutely suicidal. Withdrawal from these drugs for any reason, therefore, needs to happen gradually and gently.

Two American psychiatrists, Martin Harrow and Thomas Jobe, followed people diagnosed with schizophrenia for 20 years. Some stayed on antipsychotics, while others did not. The difference between those who stayed on meds and those who stopped taking them was substantial. After an initial relapse (which the researchers attributed to their previous regime of antipsychotics), the people who discontinued their meds settled down to a much higher quality of life than those who stayed indefinitely on their prescribed drugs.[11]

This is a very complex issue and needs to be considered person-by-person in light of their particular history. I've witnessed medications being enormously helpful to people I worked with over many years in St James's. I've also witnessed people who were on so many long-term medications that all they could do was sit lifelessly in psychiatric day centres day after day, becoming increasingly disengaged with life over time. These features were likely to be interpreted as confirmation that they had schizophrenia, rather than to have provoked a radical review of their medication regime.

The greatest drawback in treating psychosis as an exclusively medical problem is that the human factors at play in the lives of sufferers are dismissed or side-lined. Many service providers assume there is little to be gained from listening to what they view as a disorder that can only be helped by medication.

There are exceptions, and there is much to be learned from people and services who employ a range of medical and non-medical interventions to resolve complex mental health disorders.

The Open Dialogue method in northern Finland mobilises community-based teams to intervene as early as possible in an episode of psychosis. The teams work exclusively in homes and community resources to help vulnerable people and their families to address the stresses that have triggered the episode. Their research has shown that this early intervention has resulted in a marked decrease in the development of schizophrenia.[12] Operating a similar model is The 388, a treatment centre in Canada for adults with schizophrenia or related psychoses.[13] It offers a psychoanalytic approach to psychosis by multidisciplinary teams headed by a psychiatrist, and services are available 24 hours a day, 365 days a year. This multidisciplinary approach aims to encourage the user to understand and manage what is causing their difficulties and to make changes that allow their return to autonomy and active citizenship.

Karen O'Connor, a psychiatrist in Cork, and Gary O'Donoghue, a professor of psychology in Galway, are pioneering a similar model in Ireland called Early Intervention in Psychosis (EIP).[14] EIP is a personalised, community-based approach that matches therapeutic interventions to what a person needs when they experience psychosis. It arose from a recognition that there is a critical time period where a combination of psychological, medical, individual, family and social supports can radically improve a person's chances of recovery. As it involves a range of bespoke interventions over an extended period, this is a resource-intensive programme. It can therefore be difficult to secure financial support during economic cutbacks. But there are good reasons for government and health services to invest in it: evidence from 30 years of worldwide research on the impact of EIP is consistently positive. And this model is not merely for people who experience psychosis, but a prototype for a much more humane mental health service that could benefit everyone.

Annie Rogers, a psychology professor and writer who was hospitalised for episodes of severe psychosis, asks:

> How do we listen to individuals in psychosis who might yearn to speak but cannot find the words to convey their most vital experiences? … How do we receive language that sometimes sounds incoherent or eccentric with respect to ordinary, unstated norms of speaking? … What does it take, on the listener's part, to receive the psychotic subject as a subject worth listening to, worth working to hear?[15]

While it is encouraging to see people and resources allocated to early intervention, it is rare for our mental health services to devote time to people with long-term vulnerabilities to psychosis. We don't trust the power of consistent, respectful relationships to enable a person to recover a sense of Self and reduce their sense of isolation and shame.

To illustrate, here are two examples of interactions with people diagnosed with schizophrenia. The first illustrates exactly what *not* to do as a listener. The second is an example of what a more respectful response can achieve.

Donal was a university student who was bright, warm and well-mannered. I was a young psychologist at the time, which meant I felt sure that I knew exactly how to 'fix' people. Donal's problem was that he believed he was being followed everywhere by a white van with IRA men inside and that his life was in danger. This was the early 1980s in Dublin, and such a scenario wasn't entirely implausible. I suggested that we walk around the local neighbourhood together so that he could point out any vans that looked suspicious. We walked for a long time, but he saw nothing suspicious. I pointed out several vans that passed us and asked him whether any of them could harbour a threat. He always said no and became increasingly quiet. We returned to the hospital, and I brought him into my office. We compared his fear that he was being followed with our findings on our walk together. He acknowledged that he might have been imagining things. I smugly rested my case.

The next day, Donal was admitted to the hospital because he had become floridly psychotic during the night. However irrational it may have seemed, his delusion had served some purpose in making sense of why he felt so anxious. Ironically, it had allowed him to keep himself together and gave him a tentative foothold on reality. My intervention had exposed the lie in his thinking but offered nothing else to hold him. His defences, fragile as they were, had collapsed. I intervened without any finesse or sensitivity and caused him great pain. I have never forgotten Donal.

Brian was a big shy bear of a man with soft features and a gentle manner. Now middle-aged, he was diagnosed with schizophrenia in his youth and had spent over twenty years attending an industrial workshop in his psychiatric hospital. He complained of hearing voices who spoke to him cruelly. He had asked if he could talk to someone about his life.

Early in our first meeting, I discovered that he was a fan of the author Maurice West. I had recently finished one of the books Brian singled out for special praise. Our early weekly sessions were spent discussing West's novels, their meanings and merits. Our conversations were less the stuff of traditional therapy and more that of a book club.

And then one day, apropos of nothing in particular, Brian stopped, looked at me intently and said, 'I've really let people down, haven't I?' I listened quietly as he told me he'd been the eldest child and only son in a family of five. His father was a civil servant and a well-read man. He'd had high hopes for his son and had encouraged his reading from an early age. Brian did well academically until his mid-teens when everything seemed to fall apart. He never understood what happened to him but had carried a deep sense of guilt all his life for letting his family down. I could feel the depth of his grief and shame.

Brian was part of a psychiatric culture that strongly discouraged people vulnerable to psychosis from talking about their past experiences and feelings. But there were some things Brian needed to put into words. Left unexpressed, it was likely that his unprocessed grief and self-blame had become projected into alien voices who taunted him relentlessly for being such a failure.

Why were therapeutic interventions with people prone to psychosis traditionally discouraged? In his historical review of psychotherapy and psychosis, Darian Leader found that it wasn't so much the intervention as the therapist who often provoked a relapse. Psychotherapists and psychiatrists traditionally adopted a 'guru-like' position with their most vulnerable patients, which could be highly distressing. As Leader explains, 'Sustained silence from the analyst or enigmatic interpretations that the subject could make no sense of, or the unqualified invitation to free-associate could all trigger a latent psychosis, and the literature is filled with such examples.'[16]

In stark contrast to this 'expert' approach, the success of therapeutic communities in the 1960s and 1970s was attributed to how psychiatrists and therapists put themselves on the same level as the 'residents'. They treated their patients as peers, sharing the same living areas and tables at mealtimes to break down the 'us' and 'them' divide.

In my own experience, well-meaning carers (whether practitioners or family or friends) often bring a friendly attitude to their conversations with people prone to psychosis while also subtly trying to make them adopt a more reasonable, 'normal' view of the world. I have also noticed an increasing number of manualised programmes proposing 'how to think' approaches for people diagnosed with some form of psychosis.

There is a kind of violence in trying to force another to adopt a truth that is not their own. The danger of our attempts to make people 'adjust' socially is that we impose meaning on them, rather than enabling them to make sense of things in their own way. In my work with Donal, I guided him to see the flaws in his thinking, with no appreciation of how desperately he was trying to make sense of the world from a place of terror. As Annie Rogers wrote, 'Perhaps there are times when it is most human (and deeply respectful) to become a presence that fully accepts a lasting affliction and the gifts that come with *that* version of things.'[17]

Frieda Fromm-Reichmann was a German psychiatrist who pioneered a psychotherapeutic treatment for schizophrenia. She suggests that, rather than trying to 'normalise' the person, 'the therapist should feel that their role in treating schizophrenia is accomplished if these people can find for themselves, without injury to their neighbours, their own sources of satisfaction and security, irrespective of the approval of their neighbours, family or public opinion.'[18]

People vulnerable to psychosis have something to teach us about humanising our mental health services. What they've been asking of us for years is that we put genuine relationships and care at the heart of our treatment regimes – that we jettison our 'we know best' attitude and take time to build relationships with them as human beings. Some of our most vocal mental health practitioners reject this approach because it feels contrary to how 'experts' behave.

They prefer to be shielded by their roles and hold fast to universal explanations of psychosis rather than grapple with experience that is always personal and complex. Many front-line staff (like nurses and occupational therapists) relate daily with people on an equal basis, without notions of self-importance. They are examples of how we can interact with vulnerable people in a natural way.

I experienced the power of this approach from a man whose brother had severe and enduring mental health difficulties. I was commissioned to study families in our catchment area that lived with relatives diagnosed with schizophrenia. I wanted to explore why roughly half of these families had loved ones who regularly relapsed and other families had relatives who rarely relapsed.[19]

John was in the second group. His slightly younger brother had been severely psychotic for over twenty years and attended a hospital day centre some distance from where they lived. The two men lived with their mother. While the house was calm and all three seemed content, John told me it hadn't always been so. There were almost daily rows for the first 10 years after his brother was diagnosed. The only respite he and his mother achieved was when his brother relapsed and was admitted to hospital. Typically, rows happened in the evening when his brother would return from the day centre in a very agitated state. He would pound the floor of his bedroom for a long time, talking loudly in a deluded way to nobody and refusing to join them for dinner. John and his mother would wait until it became clear that he wasn't coming downstairs. On the occasions when he did, there were invariably rows about his brother's lack of consideration.

One day, John asked himself why his brother wasn't coming downstairs in time for dinner. It struck him that his brother was in a highly stressed state every evening when he returned home. He wasn't being thoughtless in refusing to come downstairs and join his family; he was too busy trying to calm down from the day he'd had. The centre was a lot for him to manage, and two daily bus journeys were an added stress.

So, he decided to try a completely different approach with his brother. One day, while his brother was at the day centre, John rearranged his bedroom to make some extra space and installed a comfortable chair and a small TV. When his brother returned that evening, John explained to him that he'd finally realised how stressful his life was and how badly he needed time to debrief and settle himself in the evenings before he was able to appear for dinner. He encouraged his brother to take whatever time he needed and reassured him that dinner would be kept for him whenever he came downstairs. The rows stopped, and the three began sharing a regular evening meal. John went on to co-found The Schizophrenia Association of Ireland (now called 'Shine'), which he intended to be a support for parents and families who struggled with how best to relate to a loved one with profound emotional vulnerabilities.

Sitting with someone in a psychotic state can be hard for

mental health professionals. Empathising with their confusing and distressing experiences requires a degree of comfort with what people dismiss as mere 'craziness'. Wilfred Bion noted that we all have psychotic and non-psychotic aspects to our personalities. Before we can sit with someone else's 'madness', we must recognise and make peace with our own.

Mental health clinicians find it as hard as anyone to accept elements in their inner lives that don't make sense. But when we learn to accept the shadow in our own minds, we are less afraid to be with someone struggling to make sense of theirs. It is surprising what can happen when we accept people with unusual ideas and relate to them as people. It often allows us to make life-giving connections.

Mary was a single woman in her mid-fifties who presented to outpatients in tears on a Thursday in mid-December. No one could get her to explain what had upset her. She continued to cry persistently. Her consultant psychiatrist, who had known her for several years, suggested she be admitted to hospital where she could feel safe and be looked after. He didn't prescribe any medications, as no one knew what was wrong. I saw Mary the day after her admission, but I was no more successful than anyone else in getting her to tell us what had happened.

The following Monday, I held my usual group meeting with people in the admissions ward. Anyone who wanted to, regardless of their mental or emotional state, was welcome to attend. I'd been running this weekly session for years. Usually, between 10 and 15 people turned up. Many of them were acutely psychotic, agitated or suicidal. But for that one hour every week, I wasn't interested in their diagnosis, their history or why they had been admitted. I had only two questions, which I asked each of them: 'What was it like for you to wake up this morning in this hospital?' and, 'What do you need?' Their lives had brought them, for whatever reasons, to this moment, and I wanted to know how they felt about that.

Mary joined the group that morning, still weeping. Another person who joined us that morning was Eoghan, a tall man in his mid-thirties with a mop of rich dark hair. The imminence of some nuclear threat to the hospital preoccupied Eoghan. He sat upright on the windowsill – refusing to sit in a chair – scanning the campus below for people who were clearly up to no good.

The rest of us sat in a circle. I moved around the group, asking each participant the same two questions. Eoghan remained on his lookout, focused and frightened. When I asked him what he needed, he told me he needed to keep the entire general hospital in which our department was located safe. Paramilitaries were moving through the grounds to capture the radiology department and ignite the plutonium stored there. He was in touch with soldiers on the roofs of several hospital buildings, who were trying to prevent such an incident from happening. What he needed was to simply be allowed to do his job. Fair enough. I thanked him for his service and moved on.

I left Mary until last because I hoped time would settle her down. When I turned to her towards the end of the group, it was clear neither had happened for her. And then an idea struck me.

Feedback and expressions of genuine support for each other were fundamental to what made these sessions therapeutic. I turned to Eoghan, who hadn't moved from his perch and said, 'Eoghan, I get that you're busy, and I want you to know we appreciate what you're doing to protect all of us, but I need your help. This is our last session before Christmas, and Mary can't stop crying. We can't leave her to face Christmas the way she is. Can you help?'

Eoghan stared back at me and then at Mary. After a few moments of intense decision-making, he stepped down from the windowsill and sat beside me. Mary was sitting opposite both of us. Looking at her directly, David asked the group to join hands. We all did exactly as he asked. Then he spoke to Mary.

'I love you, Mary,' he said and immediately repeated it. 'I love you.' I held my breath, not knowing where on earth he was going with this.

'And do you know why I love you?' Eoghan continued. 'Because last Saturday I was admitted here by two men who brought me, against my will, to a single room where someone stayed outside the door. As they walked me through the ward, everyone looked away. But you didn't. You looked at me and smiled at me. That meant a lot to me. You're a good person, Mary.'

She stopped crying. It was hard to read the expression on her face, but she seemed shocked. Eoghan had connected with her in a way that no one else had.

Mary was discharged the next morning. Following the group session, she met with her registrar and told her the whole story. She had had a brief sexual tryst with a married neighbour and felt profoundly ashamed. She couldn't bring herself to say anything because she feared people would see her as a bad person. David's words had been exactly what she needed to hear. His intensity broke through her shame. His heartfelt message, 'You're a good person, Mary,' had broken the spell.

How we collectively think about psychosis as a society will ultimately shape what we regard as an acceptable standard of care. Working with people patiently over time to reveal to them their dignity and self-agency is a challenge in an age where distress must be eradicated as rapidly as possible. Viewing it purely as a physiological or neurological disorder makes an exclusively medical intervention sound acceptable. Acknowledging the psychological and emotional variables involved should make us aim for a higher standard of care.

The 'insane' are far 'saner' than we realise; the 'sane' are far more 'insane' than we care to admit. At the heart of 'insanity', there is always someone who is not entirely broken. When acute episodes of psychosis pass – which usually happens much faster than people think – that person shows us that they feel what every human being feels. If we can be present and trust that person, we both feel more human. Recovery depends on moment-to-moment interactions where a person feels respected and acknowledged as a unique individual with desires and dreams.

Every member of our community mental health team has something critical to offer. Occupational therapists are ideally placed to address problems resulting from isolation and marginalisation; mental health social workers and community nurses are vital to extend a person's social network and link them to local resources that may support their mental health. Brief psychotherapy can help people develop ways to manage distress, set achievable goals and structure their lives. Low-intensity, supportive forms of therapy, over a longer period of time, can help someone recover a sense of Self and address painful issues in their lives. Medication has a role, but it needs to be administered thoughtfully as one element of a larger recovery plan.

Over the course of my career, I have returned again and again to that quote from Jon Kabat-Zinn about the power of seeing our own completeness. Each of us is a whole person, whatever problems and difficulties we may have. There is a human being at the centre of even the most psychotic chaos. Their symptoms may be documented in bulging medical files, but it's easy to miss their strengths and the unique spark that makes them the person they are.

In the year before he died, RD Laing was interviewed by

Channel Four and asked about his work with people prone to psychosis. At one point he said:

> Most of the people we meet are very frightened: they are consciously and unconsciously putting up all sorts of defences. They can be guaranteed to be more anxious than us, however inexperienced we are. It is therefore required of us that we conduct ourselves with courtesy; the ordinary rules of politeness should be our rules; we are harmless, and our intentions on the whole benevolent; but we have to show it. It is in the very way we treat each other that treatment itself lies.[20]

Recovery doesn't mean we achieve some idealised end state where we put our troubles behind us. Recovery is more about an ever-deepening acceptance of our limitations and our gifts. We are very poor at evaluating the effectiveness of our mental health services, but perhaps the best metric for success, especially among those with severe and enduring vulnerabilities, is the extent to which people feel a greater sense of dignity and hope when they walk away from us.

THOUGHTS ON DEPRESSION

Every time you think you are broken, know this:
No one can break an ocean.
All you are doing is breaking through
the glass that is holding you imprisoned,
diving deeper into your own depths.[1]

NIKITA GILL

People often talk about their depression as though it is a solid free-standing entity inside them that randomly takes over and holds them in its grip for no apparent reason at all. It's a thing they have, rather than the legacy of something that happened to them. As the American psychoanalyst Marilyn Charles wrote, 'It is in being willing to explore those connections that the person can begin to have a greater understanding and thereby greater control over the symptoms associated with depression.'[2]

Nikita Gill's poem, 'The Ocean in You', for me captures the sense of imprisonment and isolation that can often go hand in hand with depression. Depression often follows from a deep sense of loss for which we blame ourselves. This may be the loss of a loved one, a career, cherished illusions, material possessions, or anything we consider essential to our happiness. Loss may also be experienced as a defeat or a life-long feeling of inadequacy we've been unable to shake off. Depression can take hold of us when we imagine that our pain is our fault. We blame ourselves for our lack of confidence, how life didn't turn out as planned, for the wounds we've carried since childhood.

The psychologist John Welwood describes depression as a 'loss of heart'. Our mind fills with stories of how 'bad' we are. We become less and less tolerant of our vulnerabilities. The pain can be unbearable, so we try to push it away. But it congeals inside us. We feel trapped. Welwood writes in his book *The Psychology of Awakening:*

> Depression is … a feeling of weight and oppression that often contains suppressed anger and resentment. Instead of taking a defiant or fluid expression, this anger is muted and frozen into bitterness. Reality takes on a bitter taste. Depressed people hold this bitterness inside, chew it over, and make themselves sick. Having lost touch with their basic goodness, they become convinced that they and the world are bad.[3]

People who love us usually see through the cruelty of the stories we tell ourselves about our distress, but we can easily dismiss their consolations. Therapy can help to soften these self-accusations. Because they do not try to console us, to make us 'feel better', a therapist can enable us to step back from the ruminations circling our minds and ask ourselves important questions. Why are we imprisoning ourselves so painfully? What truth are we frightened to face? Why does blaming ourselves seem preferable to dealing with unhealed wounds and feeling our pain? Therapy allows us to see that whatever we are doing to escape our pain is ironically keeping us trapped inside.

Carl Jung went through a prolonged mental health crisis from 1913 to 1918. Its intensity was such that his wife invited his mistress to move in with them as she was the only person who could calm him down. Jung lived through depression and psychosis, which required support from both women. During those years, he suffered from hallucinations and periods of intense depersonalisation. He withdrew from his teaching work and wrote very little.

Years later, Jung wrote about how important those years of breakdown had been:

> The years in which I was pursuing my inner images were the most important in my life – in them everything was decided.[4]

Hand-in-hand with the disintegration that he had experienced, Jung observed there was a healing process taking place. The protective armour around his heart broke open, and painful memories resurfaced. Deep-seated fears were unmasked. He felt like a stranger to himself. But at the same time, this experience allowed him to acknowledge his wounds and come to terms with what he had avoided for years. And out of his struggles, a new, more robust self-identity was forming.

His 'falling apart' was paralleled by his 'coming together'. He called this the 'individuation process', and it became the basis for his later work. Jung saw this process as a fundamental drive inside us to become ourselves, 'a kind of Pilgrim's Progress without a creed, aiming not at heaven, but integration and wholeness'.[5] He took pains to teach his students and clients to nourish this inner quality by listening to and trusting what he called the 'inner voice which can manifest itself in dreams, fantasies and other spontaneous derivatives of the unconscious'.[6]

My road to integration has been lifelong and has included many failed attempts to listen to my inner voice. It's been an erratic and often frustrating adventure. It has felt like a slow death, the crumbling of one illusion after another. But I can now at least begin to grasp the truth that has been 'breaking through' as I have dived deeper.

How we talk about being depressed is a surprisingly controversial issue. Many people accept depression as a malfunction in their brain, a mental illness that will always be with them. Thinking of the experience in this way can give people a way to talk about it with others and can create a sense of solidarity among those who think about their depression similarly.

I've been depressed many times but never believed I was mentally ill. I may not have been in a good place, but I've always believed there was a good reason why I felt the way I did, even if that wasn't immediately clear. Whatever was hurting me deserved my respect and attention. Perhaps some vulnerability in me had become inflamed, some disowned wounds had been opened or some unresolved conflict had caught up with me.

I've never taken antidepressants, and people often ask me why. I didn't take antidepressants because I suspected – even if I didn't understand exactly how – that my emotional crises had everything to do with my past. I wanted to get to the root of why I was feeling so bad. After years of working in a psychiatric hospital, I had witnessed too many people being treated solely with antidepressants without any attention to the psychological and social stresses that provoked relapse after relapse.

Had I consulted a psychiatrist, I would most likely have been diagnosed with major depressive disorder. I may have been told that there was a chemical imbalance in my brain. I would have been prescribed medication to correct this imbalance and restore my mental health. I may also have been advised to keep taking antidepressants, as discontinuing them would risk me becoming depressed again.

In the USA, the rate of prescribing antidepressant medications has doubled over ten years. In a survey conducted by the US National Centre for Health Statistics (NCHS) from 2011 to 2014, 13 per cent of Americans aged 12 and over said they took these medications in the past month. That is double what it was in the 1999 to 2002 survey. More Americans are taking antidepressant medications such as Prozac and Zoloft for extended periods: one-quarter of people on these drugs have used them for a decade or more, according to data from the NCHS.

People are being increasingly prescribed these drugs on a lifetime basis. Once on medication, there is a growing reluctance to withdraw people from them. If a person feels well, credit is always given first to the drugs, so why discontinue them? If a person is having a tough time in the aftermath of an experience of depression, the tendency is to regard this as proof that drugs are essential and that an increase in dosage may be indicated. There seems to be little appreciation that recovery is often punctuated by extremely distressing moments as we process and face painful issues.

In England, the number of antidepressant drugs prescribed over the past six years has increased by 34.8 per cent, from 61.9 million items in 2015–16 to 83.4 million in 2021–22. The prescription of antidepressants to children aged 5-12 increased by more than 40 per cent between 2015 and 2021.[7]

Kirsten Shukla, a consultant child and adolescent psychiatrist at Oxford Health NHS Foundation Trust, said,

'The increased numbers of children on antidepressants, particularly young children, are of massive concern. The difficulties with withdrawing from these drugs have only more recently been acknowledged; there is a very high risk that children who start taking these drugs when very young will continue taking them for many years and into adulthood.'

'Unfortunately, children, young people and families are drawn into a culture where people believe that depression is caused by a 'chemical imbalance' in the brain, which is not true,' she added.[8]

Antidepressants bring relief and may even be life-saving to some people. However, antidepressant drugs have been shown to be far less effective in treating depression than advertised. About half of the people who take them get little or no relief, and many who do benefit find the relief limited and accompanied by distressing side effects.[9] The authors of this Northwestern University study concluded: 'Antidepressant medications are like arrows shot at the outer rings of a bull's eye instead of the centre.'

Rarely have I heard a psychiatrist discussing the limits of antidepressants, their unpleasant side effects and the significant difficulties people can experience when they are withdrawn.

The causes of depression have been long debated. The concept of a chemical imbalance as the cause of depression emerged in the 1980s with the introduction of Prozac, a drug that increases levels of the neurotransmitter serotonin.

When it was discovered that depressed people responded to serotonin-increasing drugs, people wondered if what happened in depression was that a person's level of available serotonin in the brain dropped. There was no evidence for this theory, but it offered an underlying rationale for why drugs such as Prozac appeared to be helpful. As the journalist Robert Whitaker concluded in his exploration of how the chemical imbalance theory of depression took hold, it was never a scientific fact; it was a useful metaphor and nothing more. As the Northwestern University study concluded, 'A serotonin deficiency for depression has not been found.' Similarly, researchers investigating the underlying causes of depression stated, 'We have hunted for big simple neurochemical explanations for psychiatric disorders and have not found them.'[10]

But if there is no evidence, how did this idea come to be so widely accepted? The idea was pushed heavily by the pharmaceutical industry and the American Psychiatric Association, and had a profound impact in that it convinced the general public to think of their psychological difficulties in terms of chemical brain processes. Antidepressant medications were universally promoted as the best 'treatment' for depression. Pfizer's television advertisement for the antidepressant sertraline (sold under the name Zoloft) stated that depression is a serious medical condition that may be due to a chemical imbalance and that 'Zoloft works to correct this imbalance'.[11]

A 2022 'umbrella review' (a review of multiple other reviews) by Joanna Moncrieff of University College London examined the accumulated evidence on antidepressants. The result of this investigation was unequivocal: 'The main areas of serotonin research provide no consistent evidence of an association between serotonin and depression and no support for the hypothesis that depression is caused by lowered serotonin activity or concentrations. Many people take antidepressants because they have been led to believe their depression has a biochemical cause, but this new research suggests this belief is not grounded in evidence.'[12]

In her research, Joanna Moncrieff points to a strong link between adverse traumatic life events and the onset of depression. Her results highlighted the likelihood that social stress plays a more significant role in experiences of depression than internal brain processes, 'suggesting low mood is a response to people's lives and cannot be boiled down to a simple chemical equation.'

I concede that antidepressants might have made things easier for my family. Medication may have taken the edge off my pain and made me less of a burden. I am appalled at how I behaved at times. My self-centredness came from being so consumed with my pain that I couldn't see anyone else's. It blinded me to the needs of others. Being depressed did not make me a nice person.

Over time it became clear that the depth of my depression had everything to do with a heightened sense of vulnerability on arriving in the States. My withdrawal from my family and my self-harmful behaviours were an effort to shut down my pain – I didn't need drugs to shut it down anymore. I needed to face it, feel it and do whatever I needed to come to terms with it. Drugs may have a role, but any suggestion that they will 'fix' everything is cruel fiction. When we are depressed, we are caught up in a painful crisis much bigger than any chemical imbalance.

Not all psychiatrists think simplistically about people who present in a depressed state, but over the course of my career, those with a more informed perspective have struck me as the exception rather than the norm. Despite the volume of evidence that has exposed the lack of evidence for the chemical imbalance theory of depression and the failure of antidepressant drugs to cure depression, this approach to helping people through depression is still the dominant intervention model in Ireland.

Over the past three years, I have witnessed the gradual recovery of a successful professional man and close friend who was hospitalised after becoming increasingly depressed. Robert was diagnosed with major depressive disorder. He was treated with antidepressants and sleeping pills during admission and remained on these medications after discharge.

He enjoyed his time in the hospital. It was a welcome break. The kindness of the nurses and domestic staff touched him. He said afterwards that whatever healing happened in hospital was due to the care of the staff, the security of the daily routine and the lack of pretentiousness among the patients. He said, 'It was such a comfort to be with broken people, we were broken people together.' The opportunity to speak honestly and openly with fellow residents is perhaps the most powerful healing factor in psychiatric institutions. It must be a welcome antidote after years of shame, silence and loneliness.

During the 100 days he spent in that private hospital (the maximum number of days covered by his health insurance policy), Robert saw his consultant briefly once a week. He also attended a weekly meeting with the whole team, which he found daunting. Therapy wasn't considered, and very little time was spent discussing his personal life. Although the hospital had a well-resourced psychology department, it was assumed that Robert's depression had been brought on by stressful work. The explanation for his mood disorder was that he had some form of chemical imbalance that could be ameliorated with medication. During his stay, his doctor was happy with his progress and believed the medication was working as expected.

Shortly after his discharge from the hospital, Robert came to visit me. We were old friends, and he knew I could probably understand what he had been through. I found him to be much improved, although there were signs of strain on his face. As we spoke late into the evening over a bottle of wine, I felt something was missing from his story. He touched lightly on what had happened in his life. Even though he referred to these experiences in a very understated, dismissive way, I sensed they were far from trivial. 'In terms of recovery, you haven't even begun,' I said. 'It starts now'.

A psychotherapist colleague of mine had an opening in her schedule that allowed her to work with Robert. Painful childhood memories came to light – loss and abuse that led to profound difficulties with intimacy. Their work together was liberating for Robert. His recovery was not without episodes of intense physical pain as his body released the trauma it had been holding for decades. Gradually, after two years, he began to recover a sense of Self. Or, in his words, to discover who he was for the first time. He faced traumas he had disowned for years and dispensed with the masks he'd been hiding behind.

He also maintained his medication regime and saw his consultant at six-week intervals. He told his consultant that he was seeing a psychotherapist but never elaborated on the issues he was addressing in therapy. After three years, when he had become much more secure in himself, Robert asked the consultant to help him withdraw from medication. The side effects had become severe and uncomfortable, but his consultant was adamant that he remain on medication. He firmly believed that Robert's distress was due to an illness that necessitated long-term medical treatment. It was clearly working. Why risk relapse?

I have always found it to be the case that if someone is taking medication and recovers, medication always gets the credit despite everything else that helped that person recover. Robert knew that whatever progress he'd made was due to his therapy work, which enabled him to face painful issues and choose how to live his life more authentically. His recovery was hard-won. The medication had very little to do with it.

When they next met, Robert told the consultant of personal issues he had never previously shared with him. It had taken over three years for this conversation to happen. The consultant listened, acknowledged that he hadn't been aware of this and thanked Robert for sharing. But when Robert left the hospital, he still felt he hadn't been heard. He recalled his doctor 'sitting there, surprised and slightly perplexed' by what he had to say.

This consultant was a caring doctor, but he hadn't recognised or considered the possibility that Robert had a significant history of unhealed traumas. His explanation for Robert's symptoms was that he had a 'disease', and the antidote was antidepressants. He is not alone in this belief. The American Psychiatric Association understands and defines depression as a medical problem, stating that, 'Major Depressive Disorder (MDD) is a medical illness that affects how you feel, think, and behave, causing persistent feelings of sadness and loss of interest in previously enjoyed activities.'[13] In this light, Robert's doctor can be seen to have behaved in an entirely logical (if completely misguided) way.

The medical model of depression doesn't consider that a person's sadness may be an appropriate, understandable response to some significant loss or setback in that person's life or to a toxic interpersonal or social environment that became too much for them. Had Robert's doctor asked, 'What happened to you?' rather than assuming he knew what was wrong with him, Robert might have been encouraged to open up. He was depressed because his past had caught up with him. What he needed was to be listened to patiently, without judgement. Our mental health services allow very little space for people to tell their stories and open up in their own way, at their own pace.

Someone in trouble is profoundly vulnerable in the hands of authoritative others. Being told something is fundamentally wrong with their brain can change how they see themselves. They can lose trust in their subjective experience. They may fear that any distress they feel is a sign that they are losing control. They can become trapped in a very constricted idea of who they are.

Recovery from depression is complex. It involves re-discovering self-agency, the feeling that we can do something to reclaim our lives. It means learning that activation precedes motivation. Making small changes within our reach and setting realistic, achievable goals can be enormously impactful when we feel helpless and stuck.

It is equally important to let go of any illusion that we control more of our lives than we actually do. Every day invites us into a dance with the unknown. Recovery is about being open and trusting ourselves enough to cope. It is about finding beauty in a wild garden rather than in the neatness of a mowed lawn. It is about recovering an image of whatever it was that first opened our hearts and made us want to live.

Every step of my recovery involved letting go of my defences and sitting with parts of myself that I'd regarded as shamefully weak or unreasonably angry. There were many places in my soul that I was always frightened to go to. Therapy invited me to walk through my personal graveyard of buried secrets. Mindfulness helped me to accept and befriend what I discovered. It steadied me so I could stay with the discomfort, rather than run from it.

In his Nobel Prize speech, Seamus Heaney spoke of the 'stability of truth'. Stability comes from facing the truth. Facing our pain and owning up to less-than-ideal ways we've tried to manage our inner lives is hard, but when we do, we find solid ground to stand on. Every moment we achieve openness and honesty gives us greater trust in who we are.

Sanity is always a work in progress. Maybe a life well lived is one where we can make a home in ourselves for all we've been through, including what remains unfinished. Where there is an acceptance of both our regrets and our achievements, our insensitivity as well as our altruism, our blind spots as well as our insights, our shame and our pride. A life where there are no regrets, where no experience is wasted, because each of them has been a teacher, or as the poet Rumi writes, 'a messenger from beyond'.

A painful part of being depressed is that we give up on ourselves. We believe there is something fundamentally broken in us that can never be 'fixed'. I remember a man I saw who argued with me: 'My problem is not that I think I'm a loser, I AM a loser.'

In my own life, I struggled with similar self-doubt. There was plenty of evidence to support the case that I wasn't resilient, that it didn't take much to up-end me emotionally and that I had to work extra hard to just get by in life. I never found it helpful to recite self-affirmations such as 'I'm a wonderful person' or 'I can be whatever I want to be'. They might get me from the bed to the bathroom, but once I looked in the mirror, they evaporated.

A level of realistic self-confidence is something we each need to face life. I'm not talking about some overbearing level of arrogance, but a deep level of trust in who we are. We have survived; we haven't given up; we still believe we can make something of our lives.

For me, Nikita Gill's book *These are the Words: Fearless Verse to Find Your Voice*, written especially for people struggling with mental health issues, strikes the right tone. She challenges self-deprecation and gives us a way of thinking about our deeper selves that is empowering. This is how she closes her poem 'The Ocean in You', with which I opened this chapter:

So stop trying to hold yourself back
Inside the glass, it was never meant to hold you.
Instead, break it, shatter into a thousand pieces,
And become what you are meant to be,
An ocean, proud and whole.[1]

SOMEWHERE TO TURN TO,
SOMEONE TO TALK TO

*The road to mental health can be seen as a journey
of discovery and adventure. It is a courageous
confrontation of fear, pain and sadness. A journey
that at times is reliant on the support of others, but is
ultimately a solitary quest for one's true self.*

SINEAD, Jigsaw youth advisor

Personal experience left me with no doubt that adolescence is an exquisitely sensitive time. There are many reasons why our teenage years are intense: real-life pressures, relationship stresses and conflicts in our families, schools and communities. Our teens can also be turbulent because the unhealed wounds of our childhood come back to bite us. Nature gives us a 'second pass' on these issues as if to say, 'Here's something that still hurts you. It needs some attention now so that you don't carry it into adulthood and make your life more difficult than it has to be.' Young people forge their identities by facing these issues and struggling with them. Adults can play a crucial role in their lives by encouraging their emerging strengths and showing them how to manage their vulnerabilities. However, many teenagers are overwhelmed by the stresses in their lives. When these go unrecognised and unsupported, they can take a teenager down a dark path.

I imported a full menu of unresolved childhood issues into my adolescence. My identity was a complete puzzle. Like someone had handed me a 1,000-piece jigsaw and thrown away the lid. I was a boy in a man's world, lacking whatever it took to be admitted to the club of my peers. Waves of inarticulate anger found expression in meaningless antisocial activities. I discovered just how sickening loneliness could feel. I had little or no language to express what was happening inside me. I would have benefited from someone who could have helped me make sense of my struggles. A safe, competent person, familiar with the human mind's shadowy corners. Someone to whom I could reveal my insecurities rather than building an identity based on hiding them. Of course, there were people in my life – friends, relatives and teachers – who sustained me through many tough times. But I needed something more.

Working with adults who experienced complex mental and emotional difficulties had also made it clear to me that our teen years are critical in shaping our lives. Most of the problems people presented to adult psychiatry with had begun to appear between ages 15 and 18. Many people I worked with told me they wished they could have talked through what was happening when they were teenagers. 'If only…' was a lament

I heard repeatedly. If only they had gotten help before their problems had become their identity. It made sense to try to reach people when they were younger and avert unnecessary emotional and behavioural complications in their twenties. All too often, our services felt like too little, too late.

In 2006, Ireland had an existing child and adolescent mental health service for young people up to their 16th birthday. However, it was rare for anyone over 12 years old to walk through their doors. Teens perceived them as child services where they were expected to sit in waiting rooms stocked with colourful toys. On the other hand, adult services saw people from 18 years – which was hard if you were 16 going on 17 and feeling suicidal. Young people told us that the location and appearance of both child and adult services were often intimidating and off-putting to them. They wanted a mental health support service that worked for them, with a distinctive youth-friendly feel.

I worked from 2003 to 2006 with a government-appointed expert group on mental health to produce a new national mental health policy called *A Vision for Change*. Youth mental health was identified in that policy as the priority for service development. In 2006, there was a consensus that our mental health service was weakest where it needed to be strongest. Young people were coming to our attention for all the wrong reasons. They were experiencing at a much younger age many of the personal and social pressures that adolescence brings, and a highly inflated property market meant the option of living independently was beyond the reach of most young adults. We had become increasingly disturbed by statistics of rising suicide and self-harm. Reports of internet bullying had caused widespread alarm and raised questions for which there were no easy answers. Community groups appeared across the country, instigated by families whose grief in the wake of a tragic loss inspired them to do something that might reduce the chances of other families being shattered. Our mental health system seemed poorly equipped to respond to the distress young people were feeling, particularly when it was hidden, until it was too late.

There was a certain inevitability to resigning from my role in adult psychiatry after 30 years and choosing to work with young people. Ursula said I related easily with teenagers because I'd never fully outgrown my adolescence, and she was right. But that gave me an edge. When I was offered an opportunity to create a different kind of youth mental health support service in 2006, I recognised immediately that this was what our country needed. Thirty years of training and clinical practice had prepared me to do something new for young people. The general public had made the government aware of the need for action, and we now had a mental health policy prioritising prevention and early intervention. Youth mental health felt like an idea whose time had finally come.

So, when the invitation came from The One Foundation, I accepted it in a heartbeat. But first, I had to resign from the Department of Psychiatry at St James's Hospital. I had learned so much; it wasn't easy to walk away. I will forever appreciate the range of challenges my position as principal clinical psychologist exposed me to. That role also gave me the freedom and support to pursue therapy training in Pennsylvania during my 30 years there, and upon my return, I was encouraged to establish a wide range of therapeutic and educational programmes, including the MSc in Cognitive Psychotherapy at Trinity College. St James's also left me with a deep respect for how much emotional suffering people could bear and come to terms with, given the right support and time. I didn't choose to work with young people because I felt sorry for them; I did it because I believed in them. And I knew how easy it was for any of our lives to become snagged around unresolved, unhealed wounds that could haunt us for years.

With the generous support and great talent of Declan Ryan and Deirdre Mortell – the co-founders of the One Foundation – relationship manager Matthew Hamilton, and our office administrator Brid O'Donoghue, I researched and developed 'Jigsaw'. I started by assembling a diverse group of ten young people aged between 17 and 20 to teach me what mental health meant to them and what kind of service they would find attractive. My first hire was Faye Scanlan, a young psychology graduate who brought insight and maturity to the process far beyond her years, and her classmate Mary Keating, whose role as youth participation officer was to work closely with our young people and ensure that their engagement with the project was as constructive for them as it was for us. The Department of Psychology at UCD kindly offered us two rooms where we based ourselves for the first year. It was small, but it was enough.

We needed more information about what young people were experiencing. We carried out interviews and focus groups throughout the country and asked them to tell us about their lives. They said they were frightened and worried for each other. When seeking help, services were hard to find or impossible to access. A 19-year-old woman said, 'The biggest problem for young people is mental health, yet there is nothing out there. There is just this huge gap in the system.'

When we asked them what they needed, their response was unanimous: 'We need somewhere to turn to, someone to talk to, someone we can trust, someone who will listen and allow us to go at our own pace'.

One option we considered was establishing a Dublin-based centre of excellence for young people where they could access a comprehensive range of supports under one roof. Its upkeep would be expensive, so it would need to charge for services provided. We didn't entertain this idea for long. It might work for resourceful families who could afford to pay, but the likelihood was that it would reach the limits of capacity within a very short time and have a long waiting list. It would also exclude the majority of young people in rural townlands, towns and parishes outside Dublin who needed support. Whatever our youth service was going to be, we wanted it to be free and accessible to every teenager in the country, regardless of their socio-economic circumstances or their location. We wanted to develop a model that would be flexible enough to adapt to the particular needs and cultures of different communities. Each community should be encouraged to take ownership of its centre. We needed to work closely with schools, clinics, primary care centres, and youth and sports organisations.

And so the National Centre for Youth Mental Health – Jigsaw – was born. We adopted the name Jigsaw to express a simple truth: no one support system is enough to help a young person through tough times. Communities, when we started, were full of isolated services that rarely worked with each other and were difficult to access. Young people had no voice in creating them. Jigsaw could support young people through direct contact with them and their families. We brought everyone concerned about them together and created a comprehensive system of care, where a young person could access support, appropriate to their particular level of need.

Each Jigsaw service would work closely with schools, clinics, primary care centres, and youth and sports organisations. It should never become a finished product that we parachuted into a community. As services worked together, it would not only be young people who benefitted. Each community could feel proud of what they were doing for 'their young people'.

Young people themselves had to be at the heart of Jigsaw. We started by listening to them – which was revolutionary in 2006. They told us that they were tired of being seen as the 'problem' and wanted to be part of 'creating solutions'. They didn't need our sympathy. They needed our respect, our faith that they were 'somebody' and that they could make something of their lives.

The name 'Jigsaw' was also chosen as a symbol of hope. Human beings are a puzzle. We struggle to knit the separate pieces of our lives into a story that gives us an identity. Each piece of the puzzle is important and shapes who we become. When I look back, I've become more and more convinced that it is possible to make something unique and alive out of the broken pieces of our lives.

Our small team grew steadily over the first two years. The people we attracted were a talented and interesting group, and the positions they resigned to become part of this new start-up were much more secure than what we could offer. We faced significant uncertainties, not least financial ones. I remember thinking one day that each member of our team had something to lose by investing in Jigsaw, but their commitment and creativity were palpable and inspiring. We worked hard, but to this day we all feel privileged to have had the opportunity to make a difference.

The One Foundation was very generous, and Atlantic Philanthropies came on board in year two with additional funding. This allowed us to give the early communities where we piloted Jigsaw a development grant to enable them to establish suitable premises and build a core team of what we called 'Jigsaw support workers'. These workers came from psychology, social work, occupational therapy and addiction services. They were people with formal training in psychotherapy and at least two years of working in youth settings. A project manager was appointed to lead and coordinate the service.

Each Jigsaw service has a Youth Advisory Panel of 12–20 young people, supported by a full-time dedicated youth participation officer. Their participation kept our conversations grounded and practical, deepened our collective understanding of young people's struggles and brought freshness and creativity to our search for solutions.

From the opening of our first Jigsaw support service in Galway in 2008, further Jigsaw services followed in Roscommon, Meath, Donegal, Kerry, Laois/Offaly, Cork, Limerick, Wicklow and Tipperary, along with several in Dublin. We relied primarily on philanthropic investment until 2015 when Jigsaw was adopted as a national programme by the government.

There are many people whose commitment to Jigsaw made it successful. But one person, in particular, brought unique expertise to the project that gave it substance and depth.

Bob Illback is a highly decorated psychologist in the USA and a leader there in designing and evaluating community-based 'systems of care'. A system of care is a coordinated series of community-based services and supports for children and young people with or at risk of mental health challenges, and their families. He headed up a large organisation called REACH in Louisville, Kentucky.

In 2006, on a trip to Kerry with his wife Marsha to mark their wedding anniversary, he spotted an advert in the *Irish Times* looking for someone with planning and evaluation expertise to join the Jigsaw team. It was the only newspaper he'd read that week and the only day that advertisement appeared. The fact that he saw it at all was amazing. He was curious and forwarded me his CV.

It was a weighty tome. My first thought was that this guy was punching way below his weight. At that stage, only five of us worked in the organisation. But I called him, and we talked. Two weeks later, he and Marsha returned for a long weekend and met everyone, including our Youth Advisory Panel.

As I got to know Bob over that few days, I began to appreciate his interest in our work. His parents were first-generation Irish whose roots were in Sligo and Kilkenny, and his links to this country were important to him. He also had an Irish passport. Despite his many achievements and titles, for about two years he'd been feeling there was something different he had yet to do. By the end of his visit, he was sure that Jigsaw was it.

Bob brought exceptional expertise to our fledging organisation. He showed us how to build a system of care and invited agencies and professionals in each community to move beyond silo thinking and work together in a new way.[1] But it was the way Bob approached every community that most impressed us. He listened. He visited and spoke to as many agencies and services as possible. He explored key issues with each of them: What difficulties were young people experiencing? What resources were already available in each community? What did they believe would make a difference in young people's mental health? He collated his findings and reported them to large meetings of key community leaders and service providers. He ensured that the voice of young people featured in all of his reports.

It was fascinating to witness the impact of Bob's findings. People recognised that he had captured the character of their community and their youth in his report. They were surprised by the number of agencies in their community, some of which they didn't even know existed. His report made clear how little communication and collaboration happened between these services. This meant that young people and their families often got unhelpful and contradictory advice.

This process gave people a clear idea of what their young people needed. Jigsaw could be a hub for a variety of supports that could each play a critical role in their lives. Some would be available in the Jigsaw hub itself, others through local community mental health services, youth and sports organisations and family resource centres. Any distressed young person was welcome in Jigsaw, but an assessment might reveal that some partner agency best served their needs or those of their family.

Tom was a 14-year-old whose behaviour had become a problem. He was getting into fights at school, picking on his two younger siblings at home and generally being uncooperative. The family GP referred him to Jigsaw for anger management.

When he arrived at Jigsaw, Tom was assigned a Jigsaw support worker. Rather than automatically accepting what a child's family, school or GP might have considered the problem, Jigsaw prioritised asking each young person what changes in their life would be meaningful to them. So, his support worker asked Tom to identify goals that he believed would improve his life.

Tom was worried about his mum, he said, since her father, his grandfather, had died nine months earlier. He could sense that she wasn't doing well, but she never spoke about her dad. Tom missed his grandad and didn't know what to do with his feelings. He knew his behaviour wasn't helping, but didn't know how to stop.

They agreed to work together on three goals – to give Tom a chance to talk about missing his grandad, to invite his mum to accompany him to a session so that he could share his anxieties about her and to try out some ways to deal with his frustration at home and in school.

When his mother joined Tom in his third session, she was surprised that he'd noticed she wasn't doing well. She admitted this was true; she missed her dad and hadn't allowed herself to accept his loss. She recognised that she needed to talk to someone. There was a family resource centre in that community that offered bereavement counselling. Jigsaw worked closely with them and helped her to make an early appointment there.

When she went to make an appointment, her mother, who lived nearby, asked if she could also attend. She realised that she had also been shattered by her husband's passing. After a few weeks at the centre, the bereavement counsellor suggested they invite Tom for a once-off family session with his mum and grandmother. Paul took care to prepare Tom for this meeting. It proved to be an enormous help in reducing tensions at home.

Tom had seven sessions in all, spread over three months. His final sessions were devoted to trying new ways to handle his frustrations at school. This included him learning not to be provoked by his classmates, who enjoyed encouraging him to misbehave.

Mental health services have usually kept families and mentors at arm's length. Traditionally, there was a perception that families were the enemy. They were considered the cause of a young person's problems. Their involvement in any recovery plan was also perceived to violate confidentiality. These attitudes don't help troubled young people, who are intrinsically part of a family system, however imperfect it may be. Their mental health also depends on particular relationships – with parents, key family members, grand-parents, teachers, youth leaders and sports coaches – who believe in them and may be critical to shaping their emerging sense of identity. A solid relationship with one or more of these people can be life-giving and life-saving to a vulnerable young person. One might go so far as to argue that most youth mental health problems result from a breakdown in their critical relationships. Any effective recovery programme for a young person needs to consider strengthening these relationships.

In 2012, Jigsaw conducted a national survey of youth mental health in Ireland with University College Dublin, headed by Professor Barbara Dooley. The 'My World' survey produced what was then the largest youth mental health database in the world. It involved a stratified and representative sample of more than 14,000 young people from 12 to 25 years old in Ireland.[2] It was designed to identify two principal questions: To what extent did they experience mental health challenges? What protected their mental health?

The levels of distress we uncovered were greater than what we expected. Among the older cohort of adolescents – 8,220 young people aged between 17 and 25 – 43 per cent said they had had the thought at some point that their lives were not worth living, and over one-third of this age group reported feeling that way in the previous six months. Of this group, 52 per cent thought about taking their lives, one-third of them in the previous six months; 22 per cent of the group reported harming themselves in the previous six months and 59 per cent reported problem drinking. Finally, approximately 20 per cent of this group reported very little adult support in their lives.

The presence in a young person's life of what Micheline Egan, our Director of Communication, called 'One Good Adult' – someone who knows them personally, believes in them and is available to them – was the strongest protective factor regarding the full population's mental health. Other protective experiences for young people, identified in related studies, included being affirmed for one's particular gifts and strengths, acceptance by one's peer group and having a goal that gives direction and focuses their lives.[3]

Many services still keep families and 'good adults' at arm's length. They often use confidentiality as their alibi, but it probably has more to do with a lack of competence or confidence. Families can be chaotic and intense, not because they are trying to make their children's lives difficult, but because parents instinctively pass on what they experienced, which may be the only way that they know how to parent. Without knowing anything else, this will keep happening until someone shows them another way.

We set up Jigsaw to ensure that One Good Adult would be available to every young person when he or she needed someone to talk to. In addition to making that support available in easily accessible Jigsaw hubs, each Jigsaw team works across their particular community with schools, families and youth services to build confidence in others to be that One Good Adult.

Many perfectly 'good' adults had become spooked by stories of self-harm and suicide. At the time, a very gifted GP said, 'Tony, I'm a bit scared of young people. I don't speak their language; I worry that I'll make whatever problems they are experiencing worse.' Undoubtedly, his fears echoed those of many other adults who are concerned for the welfare of young people. They were being asked to play a central role in fostering positive mental health but feeling inwardly unsure that such a role was within their gift.

It was important to acknowledge the need for specialist expertise when dealing with psychological difficulties that were beyond the scope of the Jigsaw team. But it seemed even more important to highlight that all young people have mental health needs. All young people need that One Good Adult who is willing to be present and listen as they cross the tricky landscape of adolescence. Most distressed young people do not need specialist therapeutic treatment; they simply need to feel understood and supported. A little can go a very long way. My message to teachers has always been that they need to recognise the powerful role they play in the lives of their students. We don't need them to become counsellors or retrain as mental health professionals, but to be good teachers and to appreciate how the everyday, consistent, safe routines they provide are a balm for their students' troubled minds. In the language of attachment theory, schools offer a 'secure base' where young people feel safe enough to explore their world. In the words of the child psychoanalyst Donald Winnicott, schools are a 'facilitating environment that enables students to grow into themselves and find their own voice.'

We need teachers to appreciate that listening and being fully present can be enough. This is not a small ask, but it is much less than many of them feel they are being invited to do by mental health practitioners. Their willingness to pause, show concern and hear what a student is struggling with changes everything for that student. The young person who eventually navigates some rough patch will always remember that they started to turn a corner the day their teacher listened and believed them.

One of the ways we demystified youth mental health in Jigsaw was to empower young people to speak in their own voice. Not to tell their story publicly, which risked them becoming identified exclusively with some tragedy in their lives and not being allowed to put it behind them. But to speak about their search for mental health, what helped and what didn't help.

Looking back, involving young people in Jigsaw was the smartest thing we did. Youth participation is vital to designing youth services that work for young people rather than for the professionals who run them. But I can also appreciate the reluctance of many youth services to do so. Young people can be challenging. They tend to criticise our best ideas from the moment we let them in the door. Our language isn't always to their liking. They want plain speech when we want to sound like we know something.

I remember standing in front of our Youth Advisory Panel in the summer of 2006. I formulated a mission statement for the organisation. I was happy with what I had put together, but I wanted to check it with them. I saw our mission as 'helping young people to navigate their journey into adulthood'. My words were greeted by stony silence. No one looked at me. The floor was much more interesting. I asked what was wrong. Then a voice came from the group. 'We don't want to be helped; we want to be heard.'

The truth is that designing and running a youth support service of any kind is hard. We need to talk to the real experts. When we ask them something and listen, good things generally happen.

One of the characteristics of Jigsaw that distinguishes it from other national youth mental health initiatives is our refusal, from the start, to assign diagnostic classifications to the young people we engage with. Whereas other services chose to talk about the emotional and behavioural problems they encountered in young people in terms of 'disorders', we did not. Jigsaw instead adopted a non-diagnostic approach, which is a way of thinking about human distress that does not rely on fitting presenting symptoms to a defined list of mental illnesses. We took care to capture in as much detail as possible the problems each young person was struggling with when they stepped inside our doors without assigning them a psychiatric diagnosis.

I take responsibility for adopting this position. It wasn't something my colleagues universally approved of. In the view of some Jigsaw staff, we lost credibility in the eyes of psychiatric services by not assigning DSM labels. 'It's a common language; it would make our communications a lot easier', they argued. And I have no doubt they were right. But when it comes to young people, we must be very careful how we frame their mental health difficulties. While there may be a strong desire in families and schools to know what is 'wrong' with a troubled child and have them assigned a label, this rarely solves the problem. Labels are descriptions, not explanations. They can sideline or obscure stresses in a young person's life that have given rise to their emotional and behavioural problems. Labels also come with super glue. Once assigned, they can be hard to shake off.

Commenting on research that shows how children and young people are receiving diagnoses today more than ever before, the child psychiatrist Dr Sami Timimi writes:

> Perhaps the epidemic numbers of children in the West receiving diagnoses is a symptom not of something 'wrong' that we should try to cure in the individual, but a barometer pointing to something 'unhealthy' in the society, the culture, that invented it.[4]

In 2006, not long after it was created, we held the first large public meeting of Jigsaw at University College Dublin. It was our first official outing. Theatre L on the Belfield campus was packed to capacity and we'd had to open Theatre M to accommodate the overflow of people who'd shown up.

During the meeting, I outlined our vision. We would set up main-street venues where young people could access, for free, the psychological and social support they needed to help them come to terms with problems in their lives. Young people would be centrally involved in running these centres. These main-street 'hubs' would have a welcoming, youth-friendly ethos to make it as easy as possible for reluctant young people to reach out for the support they needed, knowing they would be listened to. One of the main speakers that night was Sinéad, the daughter of an old college friend of mine and one of the first youth advisors I ever recruited. Afterwards, I caught up with her father, Carl, and asked him what he thought of the project. Carl told me he found it interesting, but not surprising. After all, I had outlined the idea to him once on Grafton Street in 1972. Our conversation on that day suddenly came back to me.

I had said then that I wanted to create a place 'where young people like me', (I was doing my best to hold my life together at the time), 'can turn when they need to talk to someone. Where they feel welcome and safe enough to open up about whatever is troubling them. I want it to be a place where they can meet each other and talk about how they are all struggling to understand themselves and make sense of their lives.' It had taken 34 years, but that dream had finally come to fruition.

THOUGHTS ON PSYCHIATRIC
DIAGNOSIS

*It's hard to describe what being a psychiatric patient
has felt like; it was as if I went into the hospital
because my shoelaces were broken, and they took
away my shoes.*

CLIVE, reflecting on 30 years of being under
psychiatric care

'Am I mentally ill?' Julie asked me through tears. Her
voice sounded edgy and urgent. She'd been terrified
to tell me what she had done because she believed
I would lose all respect for her. Head lowered, she described
how she had broken a promise and texted him. She was
desperate to know he still wanted her. She had no illusions
that he loved her. It would have been enough to know he
wanted her, that she was desirable. He didn't reply. She kept
texting. Until he blocked her. That's when she bought the
burner phone and repeated the entire process.

She was locked into rumination and self-recrimination.
Perhaps a diagnosis of some sort would have been a relief,

an explanation for what she knew had been a wrong move on her part. A flaw in her chemistry was preferable to a flaw in her character. It could have given her a reprieve from her torment.

But I did not see her as 'mentally ill'. What was at stake was not her sanity, but her dignity. In a moment of great pain, she had acted impulsively. She knew that. What she couldn't see was the broader context for her behaviour. She was facing significant challenges in her life and needed something or someone to steady her. Their relationship had been imperfect, but he had made her feel she was somebody. He was never going to stick around to care for her. But even brief contact might embolden her for now.

The pain I saw in her wasn't just about a relationship that hadn't worked. It was about an unhealed wound from her childhood that this man had touched in a way no one else had. He seemed to answer a lifetime of longing and searching for love. Her reaching out to him had re-opened that wound. She was furious with herself, angry with him and embarrassed that she had let herself down. She had to release some pain to allow her to step back from what had happened. She needed to talk, but she didn't need anyone to judge her. She was already locked into blame. Her mind see-sawed between two extremes, 'It-was-all-my-fault' and 'It-was-all-his-fault'.

For the most part, the choices we make are usually the best we can make with our limited perspective at that moment. Julie had never stopped looking for intimacy to silence her ghosts, and she believed something good would come from contacting him. Her behaviour wasn't entirely illogical. She had stayed away from him for a long time until a chance meeting in a bar had taken her completely by surprise. His pleasure at seeing her, the trace of that spark between them, and a certain ambiguity in his behaviour had confused her. She was also acutely aware that time was moving on in her life. All of this had played on her mind afterwards. So, why not test the waters? She had nothing to lose.

It helps when we can bring a broader perspective to bear on something we did that feels shameful, weak or just plain irrational. She would need some distance from this crisis to understand what had happened. She would need time to turn her trauma into a story that could hold her pain. Her explanation might not make her behaviour feel less embarrassing, but it might help her to feel more human.

How can we view what is most vulnerable, hurt, sensitive and human in a person as something wrong with them? Why do we love our labels so much that we have prioritised them over respect, care, dignity and healing in our mental health system?

There is little we can do to change a person's history. However, we can give them a way of thinking that frames their emotional struggles as an understandable reaction to difficulties they've experienced rather than a mental illness they will have forever.

I don't like labels, but I confess to some uneasiness in

criticising psychiatry. I know and have worked with many first-rate physicians who are psychiatrists. They treat their patients in a very thoughtful and compassionate way. They don't believe drugs 'cure' anything but value how they help stabilise and settle a person. Steadying people and making them feel safe is fundamental to good psychological care. I also know people who have been on medication for a long time and who see their psychiatrists regularly. The doctors they see are kind and encouraging, and they love going to see them. Both may believe the drugs keep them well, but I see the powerful impact of a relationship with someone who cares for them consistently, often for years. A good doctor mirrors and reminds that person of their dignity and strength. Some might call this a 'placebo', but that misses the point. Maybe feeling valued by someone who respects us, gives us their full attention and believes in us is fundamental to healing. Perhaps it is the only thing that works.

But I have also seen many clinicians who do not treat their patients in a personal or caring way. I believe psychiatric diagnosis has hurt many people in our mental health services. Many service users leave our hospitals and mental health centres feeling unheard, unseen and even re-traumatised.

When we see a person only through the lens of their psychiatric diagnosis, there is so much we can miss. Clinical psychologist Lucy Johnstone reviewed research on interviews between psychiatrists and people diagnosed with psychosis. The interviews were structured around questions about sleep, appetite and side effects. Service users' attempts to speak about other issues were met with reluctance, avoidance and discomfort. As a result, service users learned to say only what they believed the psychiatrist wanted to hear.[1]

Johnstone went on to say, 'It may seem extraordinary that people's life stories are routinely unheard in psychiatric settings. I can recall numerous occasions when, after 10 minutes of talk and a simple enquiry about what happened in someone's life, a whole hidden story spilt out that made the person's feelings and experiences entirely understandable. It is as if diagnosis and the biomedical model have blindfolded staff from seeing what is in front of their eyes.'

Whether or not people accept psychiatric diagnoses as valid, most agree that having one can have negative consequences. Nine out of ten people with mental health diagnoses report being misunderstood by their families, shunned or ignored by friends, and prevented from accessing educational opportunities or applying for jobs. To reduce stigma in Ireland, we have invested widely in campaigning for greater understanding and acceptance of people with 'mental health' problems. The messages include 'It's an illness like any other' and 'We all have mental health'. We've tried hard to make a psychiatric diagnosis as acceptable as diabetes or a broken leg. Ironically, a large body of evidence shows that trying to gain acceptance for mental and emotional pain by framing it as something that is 'wrong' with a person – rather than as an understandable response to what may have happened to them – has only served to increase stigma.[2] Attributing a person's disruptive moods and behaviour to an illness over which a person has no direct control increases perceptions of dangerousness, unpredictability, difference and pessimism about recovery.[3] The very act of labelling behaviours or feelings as 'mental illness' or 'personality disorder' increases rejection and desire for distance.

No one denies that children and adults are susceptible to confusing and terrifying experiences that may lead them to behave in self-destructive ways. Mental and emotional distress is very real. It disrupts people's lives and relationships in profound ways. It can alienate a person from themselves and those closest to them. If problems persist, that can be corrosive to a person's self-confidence to a point where they see no way out of the turmoil they are locked into. I accept that sometimes a diagnosis is required to give a person access to the necessary help and practical resources they need. The danger, however, is that once a psychiatric diagnosis is assigned to a person, unresolved traumas or social stresses that triggered their experience can become side-lined or obscured. The attitude implicit in how many people are treated seems to be, 'Who cares what happened to you? We know what's wrong with you and we have the drugs to fix it.'

However, when the promised relief from some highly acclaimed 'evidence-based' medication or therapy doesn't last, they may feel even more hopeless. The persistence of their pain can feel like a personal failure rather than a failure to appreciate the larger historic and social context in which their problems are embedded.

Young people especially are turning to social media that reframe their struggles as disorders. The diagnostic labels they acquire via online self-assessment tests give them immediate entry to a community of their peers suffering from the same disorder. At best, these labels give them a language for their struggles and make them feel less alone in their distress. Still, research has shown that adolescents who self-label reported higher ratings of stigma and depression and tend to feel they have less control over their lives.[4]

The increasing medicalisation of human distress has been responsible for what one of the most eminent psychiatrists in the United States described as an explosion of psychiatric diagnoses among young people. Professor Allen Frances, the chair of the DSM-IV committee, came out of retirement to criticise what he termed the 'three epidemics' that resulted from the publication of DSM-4: a 20-fold increase in the diagnosis of 'autistic disorder', a tripling of diagnoses of 'attention deficit hyperactivity disorder' (ADHD) and a 40-fold increase in 'paediatric bipolar illness' in children.[5]

The World Health Organization (WHO) is the directing and coordinating authority on health within the United Nations (UN). It monitors and reports back to the UN via a group of independent experts appointed by the Human Rights Council known as Special Rapporteurs. In June 2017, Special Rapporteur Dainius Puras, a practising psychiatrist from

Lithuania, issued a report on mental and physical health. His report was one of the most honest and direct criticisms of the overmedication of human suffering that I've ever read:

> We have been sold a myth that the best solutions for addressing mental health challenges are medications and other biomedical interventions … Public policies continue to neglect the importance of the preconditions of poor mental health, such as violence, disempowerment, social exclusion and isolation and the breakdown of communities, systemic social disadvantage and harmful conditions at work and in schools … [R]eductive biomedical approaches to treatment that do not adequately address contexts and relationships can no longer be considered compliant with the right to health.[6]

What Dr Puras recommended was that services needed to think differently about how they work. They needed a new 'paradigm'. Their priority should be to offer culturally appropriate psychological and social interventions as a first response. Services should work in partnership with people who use them and their carers. Every possible step should be taken to eliminate coercive treatment and forced confinement. All of this needs to be backed up by a firm societal commitment to social justice that addresses the root causes of poor mental health. In concluding his report, he wrote 'Mental health policies should address the "power imbalance" rather than the "chemical imbalance".'

Research in the UK on the quality and effectiveness of mental health services suggests that they are not doing well. Overall, more people are being diagnosed and being prescribed drugs, staying in services longer and reporting poorer outcomes.

Our evidence regarding our mental health services is limited in Ireland. Thanks to a very rigorous and independent Inspector of Mental Health Services, who doesn't hesitate to hold our approved services accountable, we know that they are held to a basic standard of care. But service users' voices have made us aware that our mental health services have hurt people in the past and continue to do so today. This is not necessarily in obvious physically abusive ways (although this does happen) but in terms of how these service users were not treated as human beings with dignity and were excluded from an active role in their own recovery. This can happen in both adult and child services.

In 2020, it came to light that strong medication had been over-prescribed to a young boy at a Child and Adolescent Mental Health (CAMHS) facility in County Kerry. The boy had been on three medications for attention deficit hyperactivity disorder (ADHD) for three years: Risperidone, a drug normally prescribed for schizophrenia, along with Medikinet and Concerta, both stimulants used to treat hyperactivity. He was gradually limited to only one of these drugs.

The issue first came to light in the autumn of 2020 when a South Kerry CAMHS team member became concerned about some of the clinical care of patients they were treating. A sample review involving 50 patients occurred, and the findings were deemed significant enough for a large-scale review to be ordered. This independent review, published in 2022, covered a three-year period and 1,500 patients who attended the facility. The matter was also referred to the Medical Council.[7]

A solicitor representing a number of these patients and their families, Keith Rolls, said, 'A predominant concern is an extent to which medical records relating to the treatment afforded to our clients are missing … the absence of complete records, for whatever reason, has simply added to the failures and the confusion and hurt for our clients and their families.'

In some cases, it was feared that young people who were prescribed inappropriate medication dosages may have suffered significant health issues as a result.[8]

I accept that some people in distress welcome a diagnosis. A woman diagnosed with bipolar disorder told me recently that she liked being given a label because it validated that she was hurting emotionally, even though this wasn't visible in any physical way. Her diagnosis also allowed her to discuss her pain without going into her difficult personal history. A diagnosis can help to shift the blame a person may be feeling for what they believe is some failure in themselves to something 'medical' that has nothing to do with them. For some young people who feel lost, a diagnosis gives them a sense of identity. One 15-year-old girl diagnosed with anorexia said, 'Labels aren't so bad; they at least give you a title to live up to, an identity.' A diagnostic label may help a young person to find their peers online.

Mental health problems involve the circumstances of our lives and our biology. The emotional difficulties we experience result from relations and life experiences and our reactions to them.

Our biology changes when we experience distress. Our bodies become overactive when we feel threatened. The amygdala goes into overdrive to prepare us to meet some feared danger and may be hard to 'turn off' when it's clear the threat has passed. We know from Martin Seligman's research on 'learned helplessness' that, faced with oppressive social situations where we feel powerless, the human brain reacts by lowering dopamine levels and by inducing a state of 'behavioural retardation'. We shut down our feelings so as not to experience the pain of being trapped, and we detach from the external world and feel less interested in engaging with it. Loss of pleasure and lack of motivation for several weeks are evidence that a person has major depressive disorder. But what if the symptoms are a response to life situations that we perceive to be beyond our control? Rather than our brains being diseased and giving rise to unwanted symptoms of depression, what if our brains are adapting creatively to an experience of powerlessness by 'depressing' our pain to make it tolerable?[9]

There are reasons why we remain very attached to our labels. At some level, it makes sense for most of us to explain away mental and emotional pain as entirely biological. It's convenient and greatly preferable to facing what we know are the underlying causes of our pain.

Mary Boyle, a clinical psychologist who pioneered a very different framework for making sense of mental health difficulties, believes that the diagnostic model allows us to deny and distance ourselves from truths we find hard to acknowledge.[10] Perhaps the medical model is allowed to dominate because it is just too hard to face the injustice around us, let alone do anything about it. It's very uncomfortable for us to acknowledge that we collectively tolerate high rates of abuse and neglect of children as well as sexual violence, discrimination and inequality that cause distress and misery to millions of people. It is a convenient way to explain people who crack under the pressure of unaffordable rent, bullying, secrecy and aggression in families, forced homelessness and financial strain. It can be hard to accept how much people hurt each other, intentionally and unintentionally. The medical model helps us to deny these unpalatable facts.

In some ways, psychiatry is society's scapegoat for uncomfortable truths that none of us wants to face. We unconsciously expect psychiatry to reassure us that the signs of anxiety, stress and depression we see in one another are caused by some unfortunate brain disease and have nothing to do with how we treat each other.

The fact that we can group 'unfortunate' people who break down under stress into discrete categories and give them drugs emphasises the difference between them and us. Talk of faulty genes, chemical imbalances and brain anomalies reassures us that we will never feel the way they do. They are not like you and me. They are 'mad'. This is a very individualised perspective on emotional struggles that many non-Western cultures do not share.

I believe most psychiatrists start out genuinely wanting to help people in distress. In lots of ways, society sets psychiatry up. We ask psychiatrists to see highly vulnerable people and to accept responsibility for their safety. Young psychiatrists, in particular, are frightened by the enormity of responsibility they carry in sitting opposite a young person with suicidal thoughts. If anything bad happens to that young person, the doctor will find themselves in the firing line of grief and blame. Giving that young person a label and a prescription may be necessary to protect doctors from later accusations of not doing anything.

Lucy Johnstone is very aware of how ingrained our psychiatric labels are in our society and how they drive our mental health services. She is clear about the challenge for all of us to think about our mental health difficulties differently, and gives her ideas for what a more appropriate mental health campaign might look like:

First, make discrimination, social justice and fair access to welfare support the main focus of our campaigns. Second, drop the language of diagnosis that creates so much of the problem in the first place. Third, promote the message that mental distress is not an 'illness like any other' but an understandable response to overwhelming life circumstances.[11]

I don't like labels much. But the argument is not about labels. Some people are happy with the psychiatric diagnosis they've been given and I would never want to take that away from them. The argument for me is about how to make sense of a person's distress in a way that empowers them to do something about it. We can regard someone's symptoms as a sign of something wrong or as an understandable reaction to real-life stresses. The first way may bring relief – 'Thank God it's not my fault' – but this only gets a person so far. Ultimately their recovery will depend on learning to respect their symptoms as a signal that something in their past or present needs attention and care.

We need a bigger story than a diagnosis. Something that respects the depths of a person's distress but also the survival skills that have gotten them this far. A person needs to be empowered and supported to face interpersonal and social stresses that are waiting for them in the real world. Framing non-medical problems in terms of a medical illness makes this difficult.

Recovery from mental and emotional pain involves working with a person to craft a narrative that makes sense of their experience and means something to them. They need someone to listen with compassion, allow them to feel what they feel without rescuing them, explore what has happened to them and work with them to re-assemble the broken pieces of their identity.

But the danger in saying this is that we make mental health problems an entirely personal matter. We de-contextualise our emotional problems. We must also consider the wider social injustices and inequalities that impact powerfully on our individual and collective mental health.

15

A YEAR OF LIVING MINDFULLY

Life is available only in the present moment.[1]

THICH NHAT HANH

t's comforting to think that our lives are reasonably predictable. Easy to assume we know what will happen next. We make plans, turn our dreams into timelines and imagine a future where our work will be done and our achievements will be celebrated. And then, suddenly, something erupts violently into our lives that changes everything.

On 31 December 2013, I completed one full year of 'living mindfully'. I had committed – and been faithful – to a year of meditation grounded in silence, gratitude and presence. I had written a series of weekly articles about this undertaking for the *Irish Times*. And then, the next morning, at 2.10 a.m., a cast iron stove crashed through my bedroom ceiling and landed on my chest as I slept. Or at least, that's what it felt like.

I was wrenched out of sleep by an intense strangulating pain that gripped my chest. I bolted upright in the darkness and struggled to breathe. My left arm had a lightning charge bolting through it. I twisted it in every direction to find relief. But to no avail. The pain spread into my fingers and across my chest. I got out of bed, gasping for air. My right arm had also become paralysed with pain and was losing its power.

I'd never had a heart attack, but I had no doubt what was happening to me. I stumbled around the room, banged my head off the wall to relieve the pain and fell on my knees at the bottom of my bed. Thoughts raced through my head. 'Why didn't I see it coming?', and then, 'This is it.'

A doctor would tell me later that I experienced angina at that moment. He was not referring to my physical pain but to the true meaning of the term angina, derived from two Latin words, 'agor' and 'animi' and meaning 'anguish of the soul'. I was in considerable physical pain, but the terror shooting through me was from the realisation that I was about to die and could do nothing about it.

Ursula woke to me gasping and speechless on the floor, my arms contorted behind me.

Her mind went into problem-solving mode as she considered the quickest way to get help. Our home was 16 kilometres from the nearest hospital, so waiting for an ambulance didn't seem smart. She would drive me to Sligo University Hospital. There was no time to lose.

Distracted by pain and finding it hard to move, I headed outside to the car. In the pitch-black night, I realised that I'd parked our Nissan Micra a few hours earlier on a narrow strip at the far side of our house. There was zero visibility. I knew it would be difficult for her to back it out. *I should move it,* I thought. She was still in the house, pulling bits and pieces into a bag. Clutching my chest, I climbed in, bent over the steering wheel, reversed the car into the driveway and turned it around. Not the smartest idea, in retrospect, as the effort brought me to the verge of passing out.

She drove to the hospital very slowly. I wondered why but said nothing. At 3 a.m. on a deserted country road, it struck me that driving faster was hardly likely to get us pulled over for speeding. Months later, when it was safe to ask, I did. She explained she was extremely tense, terrified of having an accident and not making it to the hospital. I had done nothing to help the situation, sitting there, doubled up in the passenger seat, muttering: 'I'm going now, I'm sorry about this, I have to go now.'

Nobody tells you how painful a heart attack can be. Previous brushes with kidney stones, broken bones, and being knocked unconscious didn't come close. My two arms were burning and numb as they were starved of the oxygen needed to function. At last, we turned into the hospital ramp and pulled up outside the accident and emergency department. I don't remember much after that until I woke up sometime later fighting a nurse who was trying to kill me. She wasn't actually trying to kill me, but the oxygen mask around my face felt suffocating and I had no idea what was happening.

Every doctor I spoke to told me I could have died. I heard this so often that my recovery began to feel like I had failed in some way. I promised everyone that next time I would try harder.

The hospital in Sligo wasn't geared up to do angiograms on the day I nearly died, so I was whisked by ambulance to Galway. They had promised me a helicopter, but gale-force winds were blowing. A doctor, a nurse and two paramedic drivers accompanied me, and I was given regular infusions of morphine. All in all, I felt more cared for and happier (thanks to the morphine) than I'd ever been, despite lying on a stiff two-foot stretcher that registered every bump on the road.

Dr Solomon, a cardiac surgeon, put in a stent at five o'clock the next morning. The whole process was digitally captured on DVD. After it was all done, he invited me to watch it back as I lay on a gurney, still blissed out on morphine. I first saw an unbroken mass of grey tissue that looked like a cumulus cloud. I expected to see blood vessels but could see none. 'That's because the artery you are looking at, your left anterior descending artery, is 100 per cent blocked,' he explained. 'Keep watching'. I did. Nothing happened. Then, the screen changed. What looked like a major 'highway' became visible across the grey landscape. There was movement on this 'highway' as some dark substance poured through it at speed. He explained that a stent was opening my artery, and blood was circulating through it again.

Health is the free circulation of energy. This is true for both our physical and mental health. Our bodies depend on the free circulation of blood, oxygen, life-giving nutrients and natural healing processes. Disease is the end result of some interference in this flow. What shut my heart down was that it had become blocked, and life-giving nutrients could not flow through it.

We can shut down the human 'heart' by blocking out our emotional experiences. We shame ourselves for feeling how we do. We see our emotions and our desires as 'the enemy' and try to wall them beyond the reach of our awareness. Life doesn't flow easily in us. We lose our zest.

The irony that my heart attack happened within hours of completing my 'year of living mindfully' didn't escape me. I had put a lot into living mindfully, and I'd naturally expected this would make a positive difference to my general well-being. This was not what I had been aiming for.

'A year of living mindfully' was an idea that came out of visiting the House of Lords with Zen master Thich Nhat Hanh (who was referred to as 'Thay', meaning 'teacher'), who had been invited there to speak about mindfulness in 2012. The chamber was packed with members of parliament as well as leading writers, researchers and teachers from the world of meditation.

Thay was led into the chamber by Sir Richard Laird, who introduced him to the audience respectfully. Thay walked calmly onto the stage. He was a slim Asian man wearing brown robes. The expression on his face was peaceful. I assumed he would reciprocate and thank his host for this invitation to speak in such a hallowed place, but he skipped the usual niceties. Instead, after what felt like a long silence, Thay spoke in a serious way:

'With love, we can face anything; but many of us have not known true love, so the question we must ask is, 'How is love born?' Without being able to do this for ourselves, we can't heal, and without doing this first, we can't heal others.

'Cultivating love for ourselves,' he continued, 'begins with the breath. When we focus attention and breathe in, a miracle happens. We go back to ourselves, remember we have a body and see the tension in our body. We notice it with our in-breath and let it go with our out-breath.

'New possibilities arise when we breathe mindfully. We discover what we have to be thankful for, the wonders of life that are available to us. We also connect with our pain, and we stop running away. Being mindful generates energy that allows us some distance from our suffering, where we can hold it in awareness, acknowledge our pain, and listen to what it's trying to say to us. We begin to understand our pain. Compassion is born when we begin to understand suffering. With compassion, we can transform pain.'

He was speaking the truth in a simple, almost childlike way. I'd heard him speak on these themes before, but the power of his presence made me feel like I was hearing his words for the first time.

Mindfulness is easy to write about and talk about, but we feel its power in the presence of a person like Thay, who lived this practice through some of the darkest moments of the twentieth century. The spirit of this fragile-looking 86-year-old man was fierce, and that gave his words their authority.

In the question-and-answer session that followed his address, one man asked him what he could do for someone who was in deep pain, but who had shut himself off from any possible experience of healing. There was a tone of desperation in his voice that made it clear his question was not academic. It is a position many of us find ourselves in with those we care about.

Thay answered, 'We need to be careful not to be too eager to change people. Sometimes what is needed is our presence and our patience. A person who has shut himself off from the world is hurting; they have lost trust in everyone. If we love them with a steadfast presence that does not require them to change, they may see that our love is real; that it is safe for them to open up.'

Reviewing the event in the *Irish Times*, I wrote that I suspected each person listening heard these words as though they were being spoken personally to him or her.

I wondered how my life would change if I could be present to it in such a powerful way. Listening to Thay had made me acutely aware of how far I was from embodying mindfulness, despite several years of teaching it.

At the time I was juggling several major stresses and unresolved dilemmas. I didn't feel at ease. I survived by ignoring myself, becoming immersed in work projects, and taking comfort in food and alcohol. My general health and fitness had deteriorated badly.

His words were a wake-up call. Until I stopped running and faced specific issues in my life, I was of limited value to others. But where would I even start? Could a stronger commitment to living mindfully help me to come to terms with what remained unresolved and unintegrated in my life?

What if I was to take my mindfulness practice more seriously? To practise for longer periods and do that every day? What if I was to commit to living a full year of my life mindfully? To begin every day with yoga and meditation? Maybe that could change things, calm me down, help me to be more present to others and be more creative in my work.

Knowing it would be hard for me to stick to such a resolution, I approached Deirdre Veldon, then editor of the *Irish Times* Health and Family supplement, with an idea. Could I use my column of 10 years in the *Irish Times* to write about my experience of living mindfully for one full calendar year? She was very encouraging.

I began my year a few months later, on 1 January, and practised daily for an hour, which included meditation, yoga and some reading. I wrote a weekly column until the last one appeared on 31 December, when my heart broke.

Had I done it all wrong? What had I missed?

16

OPENING THE HEART

You have to keep breaking your heart until it opens.

RUMI

Watching a person sitting quietly on a cushion or chair, eyes closed, deep in meditation, we may think they have withdrawn from life. We imagine that they are indulging themselves in some escapist fantasy. But people who practice mindfulness know this is rarely so. There is at least an initial struggle behind their outward calm. They may feel reluctant to quieten the noise in their agitated minds for fear of what they might finally be able to hear. They may prefer to stay inside their comfort zone rather than open their hearts. Mindfulness is an invitation to step into and feel the flow of life in us in the present moment. It is a call to adventure. Our reaction to being invited to participate may be similar to Bilbo Baggins's at the opening of J.R.R. Tolkien's *The Hobbit*. When Gandalf knocked on Baggins's door, he said, 'I am looking for someone to share in an adventure that I am arranging, and it's difficult to find anyone.' Bilbo replied: 'I should think so—in these parts! We are plain quiet folk and have no use for adventures. Nasty disturbing uncomfortable things! Make you late for dinner!'[1]

Life doesn't allow us to sit on our laurels for long. It insists on disturbing our equilibrium just when we've finally settled down. It knows that something inside us dies when we stop being disturbed and cling to the status quo. Maybe the day will come when it will be appropriate to say 'enough', but until then, life keeps us on the move. Mindfulness doesn't deny that our lives are a journey towards some goal. But it can be a powerful experience, allowing us to reassess why we are pursuing that goal and what, in essence, makes it important to us.

Being mindful doesn't require a special time and place. We don't need a cushion, we don't need a bell, we don't need silence. We don't even need a technique. Each has its place in meditation; they help us to settle down and notice things. But they are not essential. Whether we are new to mindfulness or a seasoned practitioner, our experience in *this* moment is the perfect place to start. We work with where we are (a quiet beach, city centre at rush hour, our bedroom), with whatever is happening (caring for a child, cooking a meal, digging into stone-hard earth), with however we feel (relieved, edgy, unable to sleep, in pain).

An actor needs a stage design before he or she can make an entrance. With mindfulness, the present moment is the perfect stage waiting for us to enter. Being mindful is making the choice to step onto that stage with an openness to whatever we find there.

What we notice may be pleasurable. The light in someone's eyes as they smile, the kindness of someone who goes the extra mile, a plant coming into bloom, the taste of fresh bread, our body moving more smoothly than usual, the way music can lift us. We may echo Seamus Heaney's gratitude when he wrote, 'Had I not been awake, I would have missed it'. Stopping allows us to savour moments of our lives, to be fully 'awake' and appreciate them.

But we may equally be more 'awake' to a moment of difficulty. A moment of despair where any goodness in ourselves seems to have been redacted. When our lives feel bland and empty, with only traces of the fire that once fuelled our soul's passion. Perhaps we are scared about what awaits us today or angry about something someone did yesterday. These may not be realities we want to wake up to, but they also have something to teach us. Mindfulness is an openness to whatever is there.

On a windy wet night in November 2018, I crashed my motorbike. It was very undramatic and no one else was involved. I hit a protruding footpath I didn't see and was thrown headlong over the handlebars. I remember it hurt a lot, but I was relieved it was nothing worse. I passed out a few minutes later. Someone called an ambulance and I was taken to the nearest hospital. As it turned out, I had shattered two ribs and ruptured a membrane in my chest.

The pain was intense but the worst part of it was that I couldn't move. Breathing hurt. Coughing was agony. Any attempt to adjust my posture made things worse. I lay still in a cubicle on the acute surgical ward for five days as staff tried to bring my pain under control, without success. Surgical intervention would be required eventually to bring relief. During the five days I had been unable to move or to be moved, I had soiled my bedclothes. I could smell myself. I could not be cleaned without enormous discomfort, so they let me be until the pain eased.

Thin curtains separated me from my neighbours, whom I never actually saw. An elderly lady behind the curtain at my feet spoke non-stop. She was convinced I was her deceased sister and had returned to haunt her. There was a much younger woman behind me. She was in a very distressed physical state. That evening her condition had clearly impacted her bowel movements. The smell that emanated from her cubicle was even worse than my own. To complete this 'divine comedy', three televisions, serving three individual cubicles, tuned to three different channels, blasted out a cacophony of noise. This multisensory assault and my intense physical pain threatened to push me clean over the edge. And lying there immobilised, there seemed no way of stopping it.

That was probably the most difficult moment I experienced that year, and yet I remember it as one of the highlights. It wasn't my worst nightmare, but it came very close. Normally, I would have tried to block it out. But my pain nailed me to the spot. So, I stopped struggling and allowed things to be exactly as they were. I opened my heart to what I found repulsive.

Mindfulness gave me a place to stand where I could see what was happening. It steadied me so that I could stay with my experience rather than fight against it or run away. My awareness of what was happening deepened. I felt the pain in myself and all around me. I sensed sadness flowing around the ward. People feeling humiliated, helpless, alone, searching for lost love, looking for distraction, even if it was only momentary. People caring for us and doing whatever they could to make us comfortable. A symphony of everything that is fragile and resilient about being human.

When I opened up to what was happening and allowed myself to be touched by it, I wanted to laugh. All I managed was a smile. Even that hurt. 'Here I am', I thought, 'knee-deep in my personal vision of hell, but I'm OK. I can do this. I'm part of a much bigger story than my pain.'

I came across something David Foster Wallace wrote:

> If you really learn how to pay attention, then you will know there are other options. It will actually be within your power to experience a crowded, hot, slow, consumer-hell-type situation as not only meaningful but sacred, on fire with the same force that made the

stars: love, fellowship, the mystical oneness of all things deep down.[2]

In Japanese martial arts, there is a movement called *irimi*, which means entering into the place of conflict. You step into the attack in the moment of someone's attack instead of trying to block or run away. And as you do, you turn slightly so that you're not hit but find yourself in the place of origin of the attack, standing right next to the person. *Irimi* is about stepping towards what we find threatening so that we can harness its energy and redirect it.

Mindfulness invites us to open up to what is difficult and gives us a safe place to stand so that we are not overwhelmed by it. Rather than struggling against it, we step into the place of conflict and sense what's happening in the body and the mind. By opening up to our problems, we are also summoning up the energy we will need to solve them.

Insisting reality be other than it is doesn't get us very far. What helps is widening our perspective. It pays to see the bigger picture before stepping into battle. As Sun Tzu's iconic book of ancient wisdom *The Art of War* says, 'If you know the enemy and know yourself, you need not fear the result of a hundred battles.'[3]

I suspect that my moment of enlightenment passed and that the discomfort of being in that hospital ward soon returned. But that's the paradox of our lives. There are moments when we can step back and appreciate what we have and many more where we are carried along by the flow of our lives and struggle against being dragged under. Moments when we see the big picture and others when we immerse ourselves in dealing with the messier aspects of our lives.

In one of her compassionate essays on wildlife, poet and naturalist Helen MacDonald speaks about how swifts – those tiny swallow-like birds – gather on warm summer evenings and rise higher and higher until we can no longer see them. These ascents are called vesper flights after the Latin word 'vesper', meaning evening. Vespers are also the name given to the last and most solemn prayers of the day. Swifts do not fly to eight thousand feet to sleep but to orient themselves, 'to work out exactly where they are and what they should do next.' They are informed by the stars, light polarisation patterns, wind direction, the distant clouds of oncoming frontal systems and by each other.

In her essay, MacDonald explains that we humans live in the quotidian, the everyday. Our lives are made up of simple things, including eating, sleeping, working and thinking. Our projects help to structure our lives and keep us going but, in addition to our routines, we need moments when we can step back and work out where we are going.

Swifts aren't always scaling dizzy heights. They are mostly occupied with navigating thick clouds and complicated air streams, mating, bathing and drinking. But to find out important things that affect their lives, to 'communicate

with others about the larger forces impinging on their realm'
they need moments when they can rise above the everyday.
And not every swift makes vesper flights. Some ascend, and
some care for their nests and their young. This arrangement
speaks to MacDonald about how we can better live together
as a community: 'Surely some of us are required, by dint of
flourishing life and the well-being of us all, to look clearly
at the things that are so easily obscured by the everyday.
The things we need to set our courses towards or against.
The things we need to think about to know what we should
do next.'4

I think mindfulness enables us to bring a similar kind of
awareness and compassion to our everyday lives so that we
can see what we're doing and where we're going.

During my year of living mindfully, I made a 10-day retreat
called *Vipassana*, a rigorous form of mindfulness teaching
brought from Myanmar to the West by Indian businessman-
turned-teacher S.N. Goenka. I'd been learning to meditate
for 10 years; it was time to take the advanced class. I wasn't
alone. There were 50 men and 50 women. The women had
their separate living quarters, meditation hall and eating
facilities.

On day one, I was led into a spacious hall where white
walls and tall windows climbed to a vaulted wooden ceiling.
Bed sheets covered every painting; blinds were drawn over
the windows. A single floor lamp provided the only light

in the hall. I was shown to one of the meditation mats and cushions neatly arranged in five rows. I would spend 12 hours a day on my cushion, meditating in complete silence, for the next 10 days.

I surrendered my phone and my freedom and signed a form to stay the course until it was over. In the quiet of my rebellious mind, I promised myself that I'd walk if there was any funny business.

Vipassana requires hard work. There are three steps to the training. The first step requires that you abstain from killing, stealing, sexual activity, speaking falsely and using intoxicants. That was fine. I could manage a week without killing anyone. This simple code of moral conduct serves to calm the mind, which otherwise would be too agitated to perform the focused work of self-observation.

The next step involved learning to fix one's attention on the flow of breath as it enters and leaves the nostrils. S.N. Goenka wrote that 'Breath is the tool with which to explore the truth about oneself'. Breathing in, we charge the body with energy and life. Breathing out, we allow our agitated minds to rest. I had always taken it for granted. For each hour of the first three days, I sharpened my attention on the sensation of my breath. I noticed little things I hadn't noticed before.

We moved into the third step when our minds were calmer. We began the practice of *Vipassana* itself: observing sensations throughout the body, developing steadiness and learning not to react to whatever arose. Our unconscious minds get played out in our bodies. We open ourselves to our deeper minds by tuning in to the most subtle and not-so-subtle sensations in our bodies. We allow the energies of our past and present lives to circulate and flow.

Starting at the top of the head, we moved our attention up and down from our toes to the tip of our head. At first, we took our time, moving our attention inch by inch. Then we allowed our awareness to move through the body, attending to any sensation we found.

I noticed places in my body that were tingling with feeling. Parts of me felt dull, numb, tight and painful. With practice, I began to see where my energy was blocked. There was tightness in my shoulders, down my back, in the lower abdomen and in my legs. The temptation to rid myself of any discomfort was strong. But we were instructed to let the pain be and continue scanning our bodies.

Eight days into the retreat, I broke down and wept. My body shook, and a well of sadness opened deep inside. My defences were breached. Salty tears flowed down my face and landed on my lap. My hands were wet, and my body shook. I thought I was reasonably self-aware, but when this happened, I was floored. We had been told not to be alarmed or disheartened by any strong sensations we encountered, but I was taken aback. I didn't realise I was carrying such sadness. I was rattled, not so much by my tears, but because I didn't see them coming.

In the days leading up to my personal eruption, I'd been concerned that I was missing something. I sat for hours every day, I tried to be present, stay anchored in my body and be still. But nothing happened: no flash of illumination, no profound insights. I felt a bit stupid; I wasn't getting it. Maybe I wasn't trying hard enough.

When I cried, I realised that it had taken the first eight days of the retreat for me to allow my heart to open. I sat in the low light of the meditation hall, weeping. I was conscious that the men sitting on either side would notice. But I knew if they did, they wouldn't let on. I was grateful for that. I was too fragile to handle their sympathy or their discomfort. I appreciated the leader's insistence on total silence and non-communication. These rules provided a safe scaffolding for my pain and allowed it room to breathe.

The skills we had practised repeatedly came into play when I got upset. We had learned how to stay with physical discomfort. We had seen how everything is impermanent, how nothing stays the same. A flood of feelings emerged, but I could let them run their course, knowing they would pass. I had spent my life avoiding hard feelings. But for once, I opened myself to feel them without tensing, tightening, or running away. When we learn to experience our pain and stop reacting blindly to it, we find a path through it. The way out is in. *Vipassana* doesn't encourage anyone to retreat from the world – quite the contrary – but it does hold to the principle that a clear mind is vital to survive the maddening unpredictability we meet everywhere we turn.

The retreat was tough but powerful. What I'll remember most about this experience was being in a room for 12 hours daily with my band of silent brothers. They spanned five decades and came from every walk of life. They had all given up something to be there: annual leave, hard cash, the opportunity to be with their families for the Easter break. We complied radically with the retreat's insistence on minimal eye contact, no passing of notes, or hand gestures, but I imagine we shared a common longing to comprehend the distress we experience in our lives and manage it differently.

Mindfulness is sometimes 'marketed' as a way to reduce stress and depression, and a way to be with pain, illness and trauma in our lives. It can be all of those things, but it is also an invitation to experience mystery and beauty.

Writing about mindfulness in my *Year of Living Mindfully* column was very personal and connected me with many people. I kept my word, practising every day. I tried to convey the experience of practice and any insights that arose during it. But my most memorable moments happened away from the cushion.

I remember visiting Vincent Coyle, who runs a social farm in Co. Meath. He welcomes adults in residential care to spend a day or two on his farm every week. They have brain injuries, special needs and mental health difficulties, but when they step onto his farm, they leave their labels at the gate. Below is an extract from the article I wrote about the experience for the *Irish Times*.

I pulled into the driveway, feeling slightly apprehensive. Would I feel awkward in their company? Would they feel awkward in mine? Would I say something stupid and spoil the party?

I walked around the back of the house and found everyone sitting at a kitchen table they had carried outside into the sun. It was one of those perfect days when the sun warms your skin and beautiful smells grab hold of your senses.

The moment I was introduced, I was among friends. Billy had baked earlier and shared warm scones with pride. A glass butter churn was passed around the table. We took turns in rotating the handle with its silky-smooth mechanism.

We spoke about things that mattered. 'My sister got married, I have some pictures.' ' Look at that white smoke in the sky. That's a jet on its way to Lourdes.' 'I miss my Da, he died last year.' There was time to listen and hear what people were saying between the lines.

We moved at a slow, gentle pace. We collected eggs, sunk our hands into the soil and pulled out food for the dinner we prepared later; we visited the cow and the donkey, and Vincent guided us in touching and brushing down these animals.

I watched people living between concrete and brick walls overcome their natural caution and touch creatures alien to their everyday lives. Their faces lit up as they stroked and brushed down these animals. And their kindness was returned in the trust these animals gave them. There was no judgment. They were completely themselves. After a life at the receiving end of other people's giving, they now had something to give.

With social farming, reciprocity is the key. Everyone brings something to the table, be it their expertise or an open, sensitive heart. Being in each other's company nourishes people.

Nature is a great mindfulness teacher. It can release us from our mental turmoil and remind us that, whatever is happening in our lives, we are part of a cycle of change.[5]

I've naturally thought about why mindfulness didn't spare me from a heart attack. The coincidence of my collapsing on the day of my last column convinced me that the two events were somehow connected. In hindsight, I don't think mindfulness had much to do with it. I was avoiding conflicts and difficult conversations at home and drinking too much. Mindfulness invites us to recognise what needs our attention and care, but it doesn't solve real-world problems. Perhaps the strain of trying to mindfully open my heart on the one hand while hiding and avoiding key stresses on the other became too much. Something had to give. My heart attack was my wake-up call. It forced me to be more honest. In that sense, it was the most important outcome of my year of living mindfully. I faced up to some very difficult things I had been avoiding.

Mindfulness has deep spiritual roots, which our training courses have had to distance themselves from to a great extent for fear of being accused of trying to 'sneak Buddhism in the back door'. In a world still reeling from the betrayal of religious institutions, any hint of a 'spiritual' agenda evokes major resistance. I remember lighting a candle and putting it in the centre of the floor when I taught my first mindfulness course. The group asked me to remove it. For them, a lighted candle had all the wrong connotations.

We prefer using psychological language to speak about the deeper impact of mindfulness in our lives. Psyche is much more palatable than soul. We talk about the purpose of mindfulness being to become our 'true selves' and find compassion for ourselves and others. We speak about the practice as helping us to loosen our attachment to an 'exterior' or 'false' identity – defining ourselves in terms of material possessions, titles, achievements or social reputation – and nurturing a deeper sense of who we are.

Psychology helps us to build a sense of identity and feel confident that we can make something of our lives. Mindfulness teaches us not to become attached to any one version of ourselves – to remember that, whatever we think we are, there is always more.

Joseph Campbell, the anthropologist and mythologist, says that to meditate:

> You must have a room, or a certain hour or so a day, where you don't know what was in the newspapers that morning, you don't know who your friends are, you don't know what you owe anybody, you don't know what anybody owes to you. This is a place where you can simply experience and bring forth what you are and what you might be. This is the place of creative incubation. At first, you may find that nothing happens there. But something will eventually happen if you have a sacred place and use it.[6]

He didn't mean that we shirk our responsibilities but that we loosen our attachment to all the ways we know ourselves and create a space where something fresh can arise. Where we can be surprised by who we are.

A contemporary of his, the writer, poet and Trappist monk Thomas Merton, believed that meditation was a practice that allowed our 'inner self' to awaken. This he saw as a fundamental desire in every human being. We all want to be real, whoever we are and wherever we are. But we can mistake our 'conditioned identities' – how others see us and expect us to behave – for who we really are.

The goal of meditation is to loosen our attachment to what we define as 'me' or 'mine'. Campbell and Merton both believe that the Self defies precise definition. It is not a thing. It cannot be held or grasped. It cannot bear direct scrutiny. Merton writes that the inner self 'is not reached and coaxed forth by any process under the sun, including meditation. All we can do with any spiritual discipline is produce within ourselves something of the silence, the humility, the detachment, the purity of heart, and the indifference which are required if the inner self is to make some shy, unpredictable manifestation of her presence'.[7]

Mindfulness meditation invites us to step beyond our attachments to the Ego to move into the flow of our relationship with everything that is greater than 'me'. Because whatever or whomever we may think we are, there is more to us – more than we or anyone can ever know.

Attachments to limited notions of ourselves can stifle us. One young woman I saw recently described her desire and her difficulty in allowing her identity to evolve after enduring several life-saving surgeries: 'At first, I was broken. I saw myself as a weak, broken person. Then I was hospitalised, and I saw myself as a sick person. Since I was discharged I've tried to move on with my life. I want to let go of both of those identities. I want to think about who I am differently. But my family and friends are making that difficult. They still see me as sick, and that's all they ask about.'

Psychology's gift over the past century has been to make

us aware of the dignity of each individual. As Martin Luther King said: 'We are all somebody'. Psychology highlights our uniqueness in the way we learn, grow, relate, cope with adversity and thrive. It has shown us the importance of achieving a personal identity and a sense of Self. Clinical psychology and psychotherapy can help to heal ruptures in our relationship with ourselves and others. Psychology is accepting, curious and present to whatever difficulties a person may bring. Psychology can free us to live our lives. But even the best therapy experience doesn't prevent unhelpful illusions about ourselves from occasionally surfacing. Practising mindfulness may help people to notice these illusions without buying into them. Whereas before, they pooled in stagnant waters in the recesses of the unconscious, mindfulness keeps those waters moving. Mindfulness cradles our worries and fears in compassionate awareness and befriends them. It gives them room to breathe.

Therapy creates a space where a person can relate to their experience in the presence of another. Mindfulness also invites us to relate directly to our experience, but usually alone and in silence. That may be too big an ask of somebody terrified by what is happening in their minds and bodies. I don't recommend mindfulness when a person is in acute mental turmoil. Until they have greater stability and some distance from their distress, I believe they need to connect with someone safe, so they are not overwhelmed by their emotions. Mindfulness can help in an acute crisis if we have already practised it and know how to settle ourselves and bring intentional awareness to whatever is happening.

As a child, I built walls to keep my pain away, to hide 'despicable me' from the world. But my pain got locked inside those walls and made despicable me feel even worse.

I felt ashamed and lonely. Fantasy was my safe room. From when I was very little, I learned that if the world you're living in gets too much, invent another one and go spend time there. Over the years, my imagination became a place where I could plot, plan, and re-invent myself as someone better, someone good.

According to Buddhism, our fear of experiencing our lives directly creates suffering. Mindfulness offered me a way to forego fantasy and come home to reality. This has not been easy. Facing reality as it is takes courage.

Mindfulness is the awareness that arises when I sit quietly and allow myself to be as I am. I take time to settle, I feel the movement of my breath and I listen to my body. I dare to wake up to reality without waging war against myself for not measuring up to some ideal standard. Bringing kindness and curiosity to whatever arises, I hold it lightly in awareness. I take responsibility for my life. Some new insight lands that is fresh and salient. I shake off my ego and step into the flow of my relationship with all living things.

WHAT IT TAKES TO HEAL

*The only way to understand pain
is to look at it and feel it
without turning away.
There is no shame in this.*[1]

NIKITA GILL

n 2015, I went to my GP with a severe burning sensation in my left elbow. He told me I had 'tennis elbow', a condition mainly affecting ordinary people (rather than elite tennis players) whose work involves the repetitive use of certain muscles. I asked him for an injection of cortisone – or several injections, preferably – to relieve my pain. He refused. He agreed it would give me instant relief, but he still refused. He explained that research had shown that my problem would return with a vengeance in three months or less. Similarly, he ruled out addictive pain medication, which I would have welcomed. We will go to any lengths to find relief when we're in acute pain.

Noticing my disappointment, he said he would show me how to resolve my problem. He warned me it would not be a quick fix, and might hurt a little, but it would be worth it.

Using himself to demonstrate, he took two fingers in his right hand and gently pressed them into the crook of his left elbow, where I had shown him I hurt most. He invited me to do the same and massage my sore muscles for a minute or two. To touch my pain at the point where it was most inflamed struck me as a form of self-harm rather than self-healing. But I trusted him. I did as he suggested and massaged my pain. He emphasised that I should apply gentle pressure only for as long as I could bear. He invited me to massage my elbow three to four times daily – for at least a week – and to be patient. Healing would come in its own time.

I did exactly as he told me. My pain went away and has never returned in the past eight years.

I told this story recently to a gathering of postgraduate GP trainees. I asked them how they would rate the GP's response to my dilemma. They all agreed it was an excellent intervention. It respected my pain as a symptom of something in my body that needed care. In teaching me the skills to work with my injury, my GP had given me back control, what psychologists call 'self-agency'. I left his surgery understanding why I felt the way I did and knowing how to safely manage my pain. The trainees said they would like to think they would respond the same way if they ever encountered someone with a similar presentation.

Then I presented them with a slightly different scenario: I asked them to imagine a person arriving at their surgery in an emotionally painful state. The room fell silent. Whereas their first response to physical pain would be to get to its source and treat the root cause, their first impulse when a person presents in emotional pain would very likely be to reach for the prescription pad.

Our physical bodies don't have a monopoly on suffering. The human heart is fragile. Loss can be shattering. Anxiety, worry, anger and resentment can eat away at us inside. As with physical pain, our emotional pain also tries to tell us something. It, too, is a messenger. It may throw our biology out of balance. But when someone is terrified, panicked or depressed, they are caught up in a story much bigger than a chemical imbalance.

Freud encouraged us to take the presence of painful symptoms seriously, rather than rush to eradicate them:

> [A person] must find the courage to direct his attention to the phenomena of his illness. His illness itself must no longer seem contemptible to him but become an enemy worthy of his mettle, a piece of his personality which has solid ground for its existence and out of which things of value for his future life have to be derived. The way is thus paved for the reconciliation with the repressed material which is coming to expression in his symptoms and a certain tolerance for the state of being ill.[2]

While I don't think it helpful to describe painful emotions in terms of an 'illness', I think Freud's advice has something powerful to say to a culture that always wants to take away our pain. Our fears and sorrows are the outward manifestations of some truth that may not be immediately obvious. Until we respect the different faces of emotional distress, we won't discover what they are calling attention to in our lives.

Drugs may give us welcome relief from physical pain, but relieving symptoms does not produce health. What keeps us physically healthy is mobilising and strengthening the immune system and channelling vital resources to where our bodies need them most. Similarly, we achieve mental health not by dampening down whatever is troubling us but by mobilising our natural resources to discover and paying attention to what is happening. When we begin to move towards rather than away from our pain, we begin to heal.

This may sound as counter-intuitive as my GP asking me to massage my inflamed elbow. We do not discuss how to tend our emotional wounds in our public mental health campaigns. Our emphasis on 'well-being' and constant reminders that 'one in four' of us has some class of 'mental illness' leaves us uneasy about our inner lives. We know how far short of 'well' we feel a lot of the time. The posters on the bus shelters tell us, 'It's okay not to feel okay'. We wonder if we should tell someone. But what if we do, and we are told that the hurt we feel is a sign of mental illness?

Pain is an inescapable part of being human. It signals what

needs attention and opens a path to discovering who we are. It is an invitation to come out of hiding and grow. Pain maps our path to mental health. It challenges us to face what we usually prefer to deny, disown and repress.

Humans have always been concerned with how to deal with pain. Talking can help. Being listened to validates our distress. Hearing ourselves speak can help us to see what is happening and perhaps weave the threads of our life experiences into a pattern that gives shape and meaning to our pain.

Some truths can take a lifetime to face. Usually, some crisis exposes our deepest vulnerabilities. As distressing as they can be, they present a unique opportunity to recognise what has been hidden and hurting and give our wounds space. Just as my GP showed me precisely how to relate to my pain and how to help the healing process, we also need to know what to do when we feel emotionally distressed.

We need a way, as Freud suggested, to take seriously what is happening with us emotionally. Therapy may help. Mindfulness may help. Friends, pets, exercise, hobbies, nutrition, fasting and caring for others can all play an important part in our healing. But where do we begin?

Freud described the process of healing as 'remembering, repeating and working through'. There have been many different frameworks for recovery created since then. But I believe Freud's insights into how we heal are still relevant. I have dressed them up in new language to outline a simple framework for recovery, guided by Freud's principles, and what we've learned since Freud.

Self-awareness

Self-awareness has many names, but whatever we call it, our capacity to know what is happening inside us and to sense what another person may be feeling is what makes us human. And yet so many of us live life disconnected from ourselves and blind to the needs of others. It is often in the heat of a crisis that we suddenly realise just how out of touch we've been.

The Buddha and Freud were clear that if we want to show up in this life and make any difference, we must begin by connecting with ourselves. The Buddha thought it a good idea to connect with our inner world daily, and both he and Freud used the word 'remembering' to capture this activity. Not in the sense of effortfully recalling some event or experience but more like, 'remember where you are'; be attentive to the moment you find yourself in.

Mental health is not about feeling good or bad; it's about knowing what we feel and asking, 'What might help?' Emotional stability does not mean we stay calm all the time. That would suggest someone is out of touch with the real world. Our mental health is like a guitar string that goes in and out of tune as we play. It is only by listening that we notice when we are off-key.

Our distress usually comes sharply into focus when we experience a specific shock, such as bad news, a hurtful remark or an accident. But even then, it may be hard to know how we feel because everything is so raw. And we may become caught up asking ourselves: 'Why is this happening?', 'What did I do to deserve this!' and lose touch with our bodily experience. When we bring respect and curiosity to how we are, we generally discover that no matter what we feel, there is usually a good reason why we feel that way. We may just need a little time to figure that out.

We don't have to go it alone. Talking our upset through with someone we trust who doesn't interrupt, can make the process of 'remembering' easier. People are generally kinder than we expect when we land on their doorsteps with broken hearts. We don't need someone to *fix* us. We need them to *be with* us.

Healing starts when we begin to trust ourselves and listen. When we stop fighting with ourselves for feeling what we feel, some muscle inside us relaxes. Children in pain need us to be present and soothe them to mobilise their innate healing potential. Our adult selves also need our presence and compassion in those places we have been wounded.

When we connect with ourselves, we may notice different elements of our pain. When reality refuses to live up to the way we expect it to be, we can feel hurt, confused or even betrayed. It's possible we want to deny what has happened. We might blame ourselves for letting it happen and think that this is all our fault. Blaming ourselves is often preferable to feeling the full impact of some loss.

Strong emotions need to run their course. The tears, rage and heartbreak we experience in coming to terms with some major upset do not mean something is wrong with me. Even in the throes of grief and anger, even when we are full of anxiety, it is possible to become aware of what is happening. Awareness gives us a place to stand in the middle of chaos. Attention changes what it touches.

Mental health is also about asking what might help. The issue at that moment is not how to fix everything but simply what might be the next reasonable step to take. To ask another person for support in a crisis is to reclaim our power. Our request is a recognition of what we need and what we may not be able to give ourselves at that moment.

In all of the above, it is fundamental that we feel some degree of safety. It is difficult to allow elements of our pain into awareness until we have a basic confidence that we can support ourselves, or be supported.

Noticing patterns

Feelings we insist on avoiding are doomed to be endlessly re-experienced. I attended a therapist who was perceptive in noticing patterns in my life that kept repeating themselves. He would smile and say, 'The sky is crowded with chickens coming home to roost'. In his view, emotional experiences that we repress and disown keep coming back to bite us. These memories are not so easily accessible. In Freud's view, they live in our unconscious. But they reveal themselves in patterns of behaviour that repeat in our lives. Whatever memory or trauma we buried in our unconscious (probably the wisest option at that time), we buried alive. And without being recognised, owned and integrated, our unconscious repeatedly re-enacts some version of the drama that originally caused us pain:

> The [person] does not remember what he has forgotten and repressed but acts it out. He reproduces it as not as a memory but as an action; he repeats it, without, of course, knowing that he is repeating it.[3]

An example in my own life was my tendency to procrastinate on writing a paper, a talk or an important letter rather than get it done. Not the greatest of my personal failings, but a consistent feature in my life. Because it's always easy to explain away why one keeps putting something off (something unexpected came up; a friend needed my help; something needed fixing) I didn't notice this pattern consciously for years. But in that time, I suspect I failed to meet commitments, write a response to a friend who may have counted on hearing from me and missed opportunities to say something about a situation that needed to be said.

When I did finally notice this pattern, I interpreted it as yet more evidence that I was a weak person who had nothing of value to say anyway. But gradually, I moved beyond feeling bad and began looking more closely at what was happening to me when I behaved this way. I discovered that fear was my problem. I felt strangely afraid when faced with any writing assignment. A fire ignited in my stomach. I immediately turned to other things to calm down. Food was always a reliable antidote.

Mostly, I battled through it regardless. I did what needed to be done. But my body reacted the same way the next time I was confronted with some new writing task. The geography of my life may have changed, but the geology stayed the same.

I looked deeper. I sat with my fear and tried listening to what it was saying to me. During one of these moments of quiet, an image came to me of my father helping me with my homework when I was a teenager. He was impatient, and although he tried hard to control himself, he invariably exploded in frustration at some point in the proceedings. Another quality father–son moment was shattered as he tried in vain to make me a better version of myself.

This experience of fatherly tuition was particularly fraught when it came to English homework. My Dad was a good writer. He was the editor of the army magazine. He had a way with words. Being well-read, he drew parallels between the question I'd been posed as homework assignments and some event in ancient Greece or philosophy or Irish history. I struggled to follow his logic that Macbeth and post-civil war Ireland had various parallels, but I tried to reflect these insights in my essays. My attempts didn't go down well. I grew to distrust my own voice and decided that any truth worth telling was 'out there' somewhere, beyond the grasp of my intelligence. At university, I learned by heart and copied trusted authors, believing that to be the essence of good scholarship. My Dad did not intend such consequences when he was doing his level best to pass his creativity to his son. And I didn't see how plagiarism stunted the development of my own voice. But that's what happened.

The same pangs of fear come to life when I face a new writing project, but I now recognise the pattern. I hold them in awareness, with a smile of friendly recognition, and ask them to take a back seat.

Feeling what we feel

Freud believed that if we could remember the hurts we've denied, disowned or repressed, we would be more at ease in our skin. Initially, he used hypnosis to bypass 'the forces of repression' and bring what was unconscious into awareness. In some cases, he had spectacular results with this method. But he gave it up for several reasons. He found that in most of our lives, not just one specific forgotten memory or trauma causes pain but many different experiences. And like Winnicott, a few years later, he found that our emotional pain wasn't always from something terrible that happened. Sometimes, it was about 'nothing happening when something might profitably have happened'.[4]

Freud changed his approach from trying to unearth the

past to encouraging people to pay close attention to what was happening in the present. He created a particular space where people could pay attention to their everyday thoughts and feelings, allowing them to unfold without interruption. He found that when we pay close attention to our inner lives, we notice certain patterns. And in these repeating patterns, we find clues as to what may be unresolved in a person's life. Psychotherapy requires a particular kind of silence that enables a person to act out what they are routinely unaware of, say what they might normally feel but never articulate and stay connected with their feelings as they do so.

Mindfulness also sees remembering as central to healing. It teaches us to hold our experience in compassionate awareness and allow it to move and flow. Our past is alive in us now. Bringing attention to the present moment can unlock emotional experiences trapped within us. Attention to the breath can be a catalyst for profound change.

It's easy to develop unhelpful stereotypes of therapy based on TV and films. In our mind, we can imagine that a therapist explains to a person why they feel and behave the way they do, and that person is suddenly relieved and never feels or behaves that way again. This is not what healing is about. Interpretations, formulations and charts linking past experiences and present-day beliefs, feelings and behaviours are fine but insufficient.

Freud soon found that it wasn't enough to remember or interpret why his patients had particular difficulties living their lives. To heal, we need to feel the impact of what happened – or what is still happening to us. Pain is a door we must walk through to grow. We need to recognise and feel the pain of what has happened. Only then can we bring acceptance and compassion to places where we have felt shattered and alienated.

Safety is necessary to do this work. The presence of an attuned therapist may be critical. It's also true that the practice of mindfulness itself has within it several instructions – how to sit and settle the body – that create stability. These may allow us to connect with difficult experiences without being overwhelmed.

Both meditation and therapy can focus us on the places in our bodies where fear has taken hold. These are the remnants of attempts to fight or flee the shocks we experienced. Unable to do either, we freeze those energies into our limbs and tissues. They become fossilised under layers of subsequent experiences, out of reach of our usual awareness.

In my life, I have had experiences of connecting with surprisingly powerful levels of pain and rage in my body that I had no idea were there. Sometimes this happened when I was alone. I was terrified by the intensity of my emotions. I lost touch with reality for a few hours and was consumed by terror and paranoia. I was no doubt psychotic and those experiences left me badly shaken. I recovered but felt even more of a stranger to myself afterwards.

By contrast, I have had such experiences in therapy settings, where I was facilitated in connecting with my pain with a very different outcome. The intensity was the same, probably greater, but I emerged feeling more connected and whole. I needed such strong cathartic moments, others may not.

What is ultimately healing is not that we or anybody come up with an explanation for why we feel the way we do, but the direct experience, in the safety of a therapist's office or the silence of mindfulness practice, of the emotional remnants of our pain.

When 'It' becomes 'I'

Healing also involves letting go, grieving a past we didn't have, and mourning the price we paid for what was done to us. We don't erase anything. We acknowledge our ghosts and lay them to rest. We turn our resentments into regrets that will always stay with us. We learn to accommodate them, to allow them to sharpen our empathy for others who've been similarly hurt. We respect our vulnerabilities and weave them into a fuller identity story. What happened to us changed us. But it left us with certain vulnerabilities, and we do well to respect them.

Restoration may be a critical part of recovery. Some injustices need to be addressed and, where possible, exposed. Simon, who we met in Chapter 10, needed to expose and address his abuser as part of his healing. Finding the strength took him a long time, but he did it.

Some wounds don't heal. Some pain never disappears, but

the 'I' that feels pain can change. People discover surprising strength within themselves and in people's kindness. The unbearable can become bearable. They may gradually find meaning in what originally made no sense whatsoever. That may be because they can relate more authentically and personally.

In Freud's terms, 'working through' means coming to a new way of thinking about one's life. Psychotherapy works essentially by widening the aperture of our understanding. We see the past in a new way and see different possibilities for how we want to live in the future.

There is a difference in how people talk when they reach this stage of recovery. The 'it' becomes an 'I'. Thoughts, feelings and sensations they once spoke about as something almost alien to them – their 'problem' – are spoken about in the first person – 'I feel sad, anxious, angry sometimes'. Recovery means having a different kind of conversation with ourselves. Where once there was a gaping hole, there is now a Self. And we know that Self as a friend rather than someone we fear.

Recovery is not linear. It's more like climbing the final summit of Everest. No one does that just once; they do it a hundred times. Because when they climb 20 metres, they have to back to the 10-metre marker to allow their breathing and oxygen levels to adjust. And they keep going forwards and backwards at each new altitude. We all repeatedly retrace our steps emotionally before we arrive at a place in our lives where we feel at ease.

I see my childhood separation as simply part of my history, something that happened to me. That doesn't mean it didn't hurt. But I see now that our collective awareness of child welfare was poorly developed at that time. Psychology was only in the process of being born, and it took Bowlby and Robertson years to convince people that attachment is critical for human beings and separation at critical stages of development are damaging.

I appreciate why I became insecure and jealous in romantic relationships. We only ever know how vulnerable we are when we are in love. When I found someone who loved me, I became terrified of losing that intimacy. A part of me was right to be terrified because I'd experienced first-hand how devastating that could be, and I didn't want to go there again.

My experiences gave my empathy an edge. I felt in my bones the pain of some people with whom my own issues resonated. This encouraged me to deal with my demons rather than allow them to impede my work with people in any way.

Both therapy and mindfulness invite us to experience our lives so we can live more freely. Therapy allows us to unsnag our emotions and befriend our alienated selves. Therapy restores a fuller sense of Self. Mindfulness respects that Self but invites us to step beyond it into the flow of our relationship with something even greater.

TOWARDS A MORE HUMANE MENTAL
HEALTH SERVICE

*I eventually plucked up the courage to ask for a
referral to our local mental health service, where
I told them my story. And they told me what was
wrong with me. My feelings were not 'normal'; I had a
mental illness and required medication.*

A WOMAN IN HER MID-FORTIES

The Covid-19 pandemic hit Sarah hard. Lots of issues in her life got stirred up. Being alone and isolated didn't help. When things got too much, she was admitted to a psychiatric hospital because she felt unsafe alone. She and I had worked together a long time ago, and she texted to let me know. It was supposed to be a brief admission, but after two months, she was still in the hospital. I arranged to visit.

When I did, it was a warm September day, and we sat in the garden on a long bench. She looked well, but she said her self-confidence was almost non-existent. She had made friends with one or two nurses and some people on her ward. But she wasn't getting on so well with her psychiatric team. 'This is a safe place, but it's not a caring place,' she said. Rightly or wrongly, she had the impression that they were disappointed in her and blamed her in some ways for being so disoriented. They had not been able to make sense of why she had relapsed. I asked her if anything had helped, and she told me a story.

One late Friday afternoon, at the end of another frustrating week, her consultant passed by her room on her way home. Then she circled back, entered Sarah's room, sat on the bed and chatted with her. The two women were very close in age. It sounded like they had a spontaneous, genuine conversation. The consultant said something to the effect, 'I know this is a tough time for you. We also find it tough because we don't know what's wrong and are unsure what to do. Whatever you're going through is psychological.' She went on to say that if it were a straightforward depression or psychosis, she could at least give her medicine, but there was no obvious intervention she could make in her case. The psychologist on the team had seen Sarah for six sessions of CBT, but it hadn't helped her much.

This interlude was memorable to Sarah because the psychiatrist had never spoken to her in this way. She felt like it was a caring conversation between people who were equals. It was entirely unscheduled and lasted probably twenty minutes. There was no need for the consultant to return, but she did. Because she cared. The consultant had no idea how much her kindness meant to Sarah. If asked, I suspect she would not rate it as important in the overall 'treatment' plan. And yet this was a significant event for Sarah during her time in hospital. She had chosen to share that instant of spontaneous care when I'd asked her if anything had helped. It was a moment where she felt respected and understood. A conversation that had given her hope. There is more to Sarah's experience, but her description of her spontaneous encounter with her consultant psychiatrist cuts right to the heart of what is 'insane' about our mental health system. We prioritise the more technical aspects of care – diagnosis, medication, interventions – while all our evidence tells us that the non-technical aspects of care – presence, genuineness, meaning and solidarity – are what help people to recover.

Mental health services need to become places where relationships, meaning and values are given priority over more biomedical approaches to healing. In a large study of users' views of services, Rogers found that many did not value the technical expertise of mental health professionals as much as they did the human aspects of their encounters, such as being listened to, taken seriously, and treated with dignity, kindness and respect.

People get better because they feel cared for, listened to and taken seriously, and when they are given practical help to resolve real-world problems. Genuine care mobilises a sense of hope and meaning, which is fundamental to recovery. Despite the growing dissatisfaction among service users and a sense of demoralisation among many younger psychiatrists with the dominance of this 'technical' approach to care, the majority in the profession are holding fast to a biomedical model of human suffering where the emphasis is on 'the mastery of technology to allow progress in the development of brain research, genetics, pharmacology and neuroradiology'.[1]

Psychiatry is being challenged today because its take on mental and emotional pain has led to the medicalisation of everyday life, which, in turn, is associated with expanding markets for psychotropic medications.

But research shows that people gain limited benefits from antidepressant medication, electroconvulsive therapy (ECT) and the more technical features of CBT. Drugs may help, but not in the way drug companies have tried to market their benefits. They do not correct supposed chemical imbalances. Studies have shown that 'sham ECT' (that is, ECT administered without an actual electric shock) is equally as effective as actual ECT, if not more so. CBT claims to work by correcting our faulty beliefs, which are believed to cause depression.; however, several studies have shown that most of CBT's specific 'cognitive' features can be excluded from therapy without adversely affecting outcomes.

A review of over 5,000 psychotherapy cases treated in various National Health Service (NHS) settings in the UK found that the most significant factor in whether or not the person found therapy helpful or effective was the quality of their relationship with their therapist. Naturally, we have to be careful in how we interpret these findings. In some ways, it's like the researchers investigated 5,000 soups and found that the common ingredient in all soups was water. It would be unlikely that we would settle for water alone when we order soup. Such findings can give the impression that merely 'chatting' with a staff member is enough to reverse the impact of childhood wounds that people have carried for years. I've had wonderful relationships that did not resolve my emotional problems. My psychological wounds were elusive and out of reach of my conscious awareness. I needed disciplined and skilful therapy to bring what was hidden into the light and enable me to face it safely. The pain of those who turn to mental health services for help is often as intense and complex. Relationships where service users feel heard and respected are fundamental to recovery. People who turn to us for help deserve a caring, supportive environment and also access to someone who knows their way around the human psyche.

I know people who have been let down by our mental health services, particularly those who spent several periods in a psychiatric hospital. Nothing abusive happened to them, but they felt their most basic needs and concerns were not respected. Family interventions that could have achieved mutual understanding and respect weren't considered, traumas were left unacknowledged and unresolved and no consideration was given to their practical concerns, such as financial debt or social isolation. Opportunities were missed that could have made a real difference in their lives. Instead, the same stresses that triggered an emotional crisis were waiting for them at the hospital gates on discharge.

In their challenge to psychiatry to adopt a different approach to mental health, Pat Bracken and more than 30 other psychiatrists proposed that the profession move beyond the current 'technical' model of care and bring their work into line with the evidence for what counts most in recovery. Their paper concludes:

> The evidence is becoming clear that to improve outcomes for our patients, we must focus more on contexts, relationships and the creation of services where the promotion of dignity, respect, meaning and engagement are prioritised. We must become more comfortable with cultural diversity, user empowerment and the importance of peer support. The evidence base is telling us that we need a radical shift in our understanding of what is needed at the heart (and perhaps soul) of mental health practice.[2]

The importance of trauma-informed care

How can we shift from a disease model that explains our distress in terms of something wrong with us to a different paradigm that sees the majority of mental health difficulties in terms of something that has happened to us, and may still be happening? One encouraging development has emerged from our growing awareness of trauma. Through making their voices heard, survivors of trauma have made us keenly aware of the lasting emotional impact it can have on all our lives. Our mental health suffers, as does our ability to make the most of educational and social opportunities. The very close correlation between childhood experiences of trauma and physical illness in adulthood has made us realise that human beings don't easily recover from trauma.

The adverse childhood experiences (ACE) study is one of the largest investigations of childhood abuse and neglect, household challenges, and later-life health and well-being. The original ACE study was conducted at Kaiser Permanente (in the US) from 1995 to 1997.

The results of this survey made it very clear that people don't grow out from trauma as much as they grow *into* it. As the author of *The Body Keeps the Score,* Bessel van der Kolk, writes:

> The memory of trauma is encoded in the viscera, in heartbreaking and gut-wrenching emotions, in autoimmune disorders and in skeletal/muscular problems ... Trauma is not the story of something that happened back then. It's the current imprint of that pain, horror, and fear living inside people.[3]

Trauma is not a disease or a disorder, it is a wound. Not a physical injury but a wound to the psyche, to the soul.

The wounds of trauma are what we all have in common. They unite us. But they can also divide us and keep us apart from each other. We wear cloaks of shame because we are embarrassed by our scars. We wear masks to hide from each other. We pretend we are fine.

Trauma refers to what happens inside us when we experience intensely distressing events – natural disasters, rape, a road traffic accident. These experiences are described as traumatic because nothing had prepared us for them; we can't take them in. They are life changing.

But trauma can also result from experiences that may be less obvious but no less wounding: growing up in a home where the threat of something bad happening is always in the air; experiences of loss, separation and neglect; extended periods of isolation and loneliness.

All of these experiences provoke powerful emotions inside us. Normally, when we are threatened, we seek closeness to someone with whom we feel safe, fight back or try to escape what is happening. But when we can't access safety, fight back or escape, we freeze. We take the intense feelings that have been churned up inside us and lock them into our muscles and tissues. We cope by shutting down the memory of what happened. We avoid people and places that might reawaken those memories. We don't want to re-live that pain ever again.

Trauma in childhood often leaves a deep longing to feel needed, validated and valued. These children grow up with a great deal of confusion regarding what they deserve and what they don't deserve. They may become overly compliant and desperate for approval.

If their wounds remain unhealed as they grow into adulthood, they may turn to self-harm, promiscuity and addictions to regulate their chaotic inner life. The actor and comedian Russell Brand spoke about how he dealt with trauma through substance abuse: 'Drugs and alcohol are not my problem,' he wrote. 'Reality is my problem, drugs and alcohol are my solution.'

Unhealed remnants of trauma are like homeless orphans who stand outside our houses looking in the window at our happy 'normal' lives and wishing they could be part of it. But we don't allow them in because we are embarrassed by our wounds. We fear they'll mess everything up. We pull the curtains and hope they will go away. But they don't. They rattle the window frames to remind us they are still there.

Trauma shatters our trust in ourselves and often in others. We dread 'bad' things happening because we know that they can. We are slow to trust because we know how cruel other people can be. We remain alert to any threat and are primed to fight back. We have flashbacks, nightmares and shudders of anxiety because our bodies need a way to release excessive fear.

Traumatic memories surface when it's safe, but they can be triggered by experiences in the present that remind us of what happened. Whenever they emerge, they are usually still raw. We need to be in a place where we can look after them. We need a community with whom we feel safe. We need people who ensure we eat, sleep and care for ourselves.

Trauma has given us a new way of viewing emotional and mental pain. Since the incidence of trauma in people who turn to mental health services is much higher than in the general population, it has become policy for these services to shift to using a 'trauma-informed' approach with service users. The literature on trauma has made us more aware of how easily – often unintentionally – people can be 're-traumatised' by experiences in our mental health services.

Sarah's experience of psychiatric in-patient care was that of being re-traumatised. She describes this below in an email written several months after her discharge. She wanted me to give an honest and full account of her overall experience – the bad, as well as the good. While her words do not make for easy reading, it is important that we hear them and learn from them if we are serious about wanting to make our care systems 'trauma-sensitive'. I suspect she isn't alone in finding our services hurtful and disabling. Recalling that afternoon when her consultant stopped by her room to chat with her, Sarah wrote:

> That afternoon, I remember the overwhelming feeling of someone finally having understood broadly what was wrong with me and sitting with me. 'This is psychological,' she said, 'and it's not easy at all to understand, it's very

difficult, we don't have an answer', or words to that effect.
And it seemed like a conversation of equals.

Our humane conversation had given me hope. After
many weeks in the hospital, seeming to get worse, I had
begun to trust her because I was so desperate to trust
someone. Her relatable conversation had spoken to a
part of me that knew I had done a lot of psychological
work in my life and, therefore, I would be able to find
my way, difficult and all as she said it was.

But then that's where the hope stopped. I got no help
understanding my 'psychological' diagnosis because I
was left alone very soon after.

Over the following weeks, I cried each time I saw
her. I was lost and getting more lost. I had no idea how
to help myself – I was really, really stuck. No medication
could help. No therapy would be provided – just a
continuation of an overly simplistic formulation by
a psychologist. No support to help me to understand
what was going on with me. No hint of unravelling
anything with me or talking safely and supportively
about the litany of things I was told I was doing wrong
in my life. Their advice was to keep going to art and
pottery and the garden and using the 'decider skills'!
They kept telling me that I was doing the right things.
But I was getting worse.

Once, I descended into inconsolable crying at the
weekly ward round, and the team just looked at me and

offered no help. Another day the consultant shouted at me – 'Look at you, just look at you,' as if to say, 'Look at how pathetic you are, you're a hopeless case,' and she picked up her keys and stormed out of the room.

I had no idea what she thought of me, really. Whatever humanity she showed in that earlier conversation had disappeared. It was like being kicked on the ground and left there. I still feel very hurt by it all.

As patients, we don't need people in power to mistreat us. We don't need them churning out diagnosis after diagnosis. The longer you're in hospital, the more diagnoses you are given. When the team doesn't know what to do, you get asked to do more questionnaires and tests to learn more about what else is 'wrong' with you. That's not helpful. Because a diagnosis isn't a solution, it's another label about how 'imperfect' I am. Unless the hospital provides honest and genuine support to help a person understand themselves as an individual, not a diagnosis, then the whole system doesn't work.

In my experience, under the 'care' of that consultant, I wasn't treated as an equal. As time passed, she created a list of faults that I had - it went from bipolar to 'It's all psychological', to 'You have an emotionally unstable personality disorder', and then, 'You have an obsessive-compulsive personality disorder.' Finally, she referred to my earlier admission to hospital: 'The notes from your first admission stated that you had a personality disorder. It's been there all the time; there's proof in your file from 26 years ago! How have you not known this?'

The 'We're right' and 'You're wrong' approaches got to me. On the one hand, they implied they knew exactly what was wrong with me, but on the other hand, they implied that I had to figure out how to get well because they couldn't help with that. That was my job, I had to take responsibility.

As patients, we need a lot more in our services than a glint of hope from one afternoon when a conversation with a consultant psychiatrist felt relatable. We need so much more than that – because that's not good enough, that's not good enough at all.

Over my career, I've witnessed the publication of three national mental health policies. In *Planning for the Future* (1984), the word trauma is not mentioned; in *A Vision For Change* (2006), it is mentioned three times, mainly in connection with general hospital settings. The most recent mental health policy in Ireland, *Sharing The Vision* (2020), mentions trauma 27 times and prioritises moving towards a trauma-informed mental health service. This is a welcome 'top-down' strategy to improve our mental health services for all those who turn to them for support.

However, change needs more than 'top-down' initiatives. It will only happen when these are accompanied by 'bottom-up' initiatives. Sarah's experience was one of not being listened to and not being given the encouragement and the skills to re-discover her inner strength and make sense of what had happened to her. We need to listen to the feedback of those who use our services and are hurt by them.

This is not to deny improvements in our mental health services. But many of these positive changes have come about through our willingness to listen to the voices of people who have needed and used our services. There is a growing service user movement worldwide, including in this country: for example, The Critical Voices Network, Hearing Voices Network and Mad in Ireland. They share a common aim of wanting society and services to see the experiences of distress and alienation in human rather than medical terms.

Recovery colleges are also gaining traction in Ireland. Working hand in hand with people like Sarah who've survived less-than-ideal experiences of our health system, they aim to create 'a culture of recovery in the community by providing transformative educational courses, resources and creative spaces accessible to anyone who wants to learn about mental health recovery'. These colleges provide mutually respectful spaces where both personal and professional skills are valued and where 'students' – rather than 'patients' or 'service users' – are encouraged to build on their inherent strengths and resources.

Trauma-informed care is a complex idea that has many implications. We can't undo what happened, but we can create a context that allows a person to gradually come to terms with difficult experiences. Being trauma-informed means asking ourselves, 'To what extent are the environments we offer safe? Are they places where people experience some degree of predictability and control? To what extent are the relationships we offer safe? Do they enable someone who may be extremely sensitive to criticism or rejection to trust us?'

Traumatised people can have difficulty knowing what is going on in their bodies. They often can't tell what is upsetting them. They either react to stress by becoming 'spaced out' or excessively angry. Being trauma-informed means reflecting on our behaviour as mental health professionals and asking, 'Do we make it safe for a person to come to terms with what happened to them? Or might this service unintentionally add to their sense of uneasiness? Are we aware of times when we may be unintentionally intrusive or overly detached? To what extent can we sit with pain without filling awkward silences? To what extent do we allow people to reflect on what happened to them in their own time?' Essentially, it means a different way of thinking about the problems for which people seek help. Rather than asking, 'What is wrong with you?', being trauma-sensitive means asking, 'What happened to you?'

We sometimes think of trauma as something that needs to be talked out at length, at least for the full 45 to 50 minutes of a therapy session. But that's not usually what people who've been traumatised need. In his book with Oprah Winfrey, *What Happened to You?*, Bruce Perry, a child psychiatrist and neuroscientist, recounts a story that captures what matters to people who've been traumatised. On the one hand, it illustrates how little we need to do, and on the other hand, it shows how healing even simple encounters can be.

A three-year-old boy was sitting with his mother when there was a home invasion. His mother was killed as she sat beside him. Bruce Perry saw this boy professionally to support him in coming to terms with the trauma. After six weeks, the boy's father phoned to say that the boy had become suicidal. 'He just tried to kill himself,' he said.

Bruce thought this strange. He listened as the father told him the boy had run into traffic after they had been talking about missing Mom. On closer scrutiny, it emerged that they had both been shopping in a local supermarket, with the boy sitting in the cart as they moved through the aisles. When they reached the checkout, he was at eye level with the cashier. She had the same hair colour as his mother and was a similar age. He looked at her and said to her, 'My mom's dead. She was killed.' The cashier replied, 'Oh honey, I'm so sorry.' And that was it.

His dad, a very caring father, heard this exchange and decided that his son needed to talk about the trauma he had experienced. As they walked to the car, he tried to encourage him to say more. 'It's ok to talk about her,' he said. 'I miss her too.' He spoke gently, reminding the boy of their loving moments with 'Mom'. As he kept talking, his son became more addled. By the time they reached the car, the little boy jumped out of the cart and ran around the car park into oncoming traffic.

Perry explains that when the little boy spoke to the cashier, he was in control. But he wasn't in control when the dad tried to coax him to talk about his mom. The only thing he could do to regain control was to jump out of the cart and escape from his dad. With the cashier, he said as much as he could say in that moment – no more than five seconds worth – and she gave him just the right amount of reassurance. She neither ignored him nor overreacted. Coming to terms with trauma takes time. Perry says it is not protracted sessions of self-disclosure that heal the wounds of trauma, but rather 'controllable, brief revisits that allow our highly sensitised nervous systems to slowly, painfully "reset" themselves'. The cashier responded with the right 'dose' of listening and validation. The dad, without meaning to, pushed the boy beyond a point where the child felt in control of the situation. Moments of presence are powerful, and the correct 'dosage' of presence may be a matter of seconds or minutes. As Perry wrote, 'It is the [right] therapeutic dosing that really leads to healing. Moments. Fully present, powerful but brief.'[4] It can also be the case that people who've been traumatised speak too much about what has happened in a way that the listener finds hard to take. The psychoanalyst Jacques Lacan calls this 'empty speech', a story that feels so detached from the traumatised person that it feels devoid of meaning and emotion. One of the ways we see this is when a person with trauma speaks about horrific experiences in a detached, matter-of-fact way. As they speak without any apparent filter, we can become overwhelmed by the emotions their story triggers. They may need us to contain them without appearing to be unwilling to hear what they need to say. They need to know they don't need to say everything in this meeting. That there will be another time, that they've done enough good work for one day.

One young woman I met socially asked if she could tell me something about her growing up in the care of the State. When she spoke, she recounted one sexually violent experience after another in an emotionally detached way. My body tensed with each new horror. I sensed she lacked a natural filter that might have allowed her to register when she had shared enough. I interrupted her flow and commented gently that she had clearly suffered, but my concern was about what it was like to share something so intimate with a stranger. I invited her to take a moment to check how she felt in her body. She paused, said she was OK, but asked if she could read me some poems she'd written, instead of describing all the bad things that had happened to her. Her poetry was evocative but less disturbing than her narrative. In writing about her experiences, she had been able to step back from them emotionally and reflect on them symbolically, allowing both herself and her listener to hear her.

Seeing distress through a trauma-informed lens helps move our thinking from chasing symptoms to an awareness that there is history and hurt behind those symptoms. Not that we should go digging for trauma, but that we should be aware that there is a need to 'tread softly' because we may be stepping on wounds that require a particular kind of sensitivity.

A more humane mental health service

We need more resources, but we don't necessarily need more of the same.

We can build a humane mental health service from the inside out, and it has to begin with each of us. We need to look at our own lives and be honest about what has hurt and helped us. What interventions were life-giving, and what kind of behaviours kept us stuck? We each have a story, one that has taught us much that can be of help to others.

A humane mental health service is one where people in distress form real relationships with those who care for them, allowing them to face their experiences and come to a deeper understanding of themselves, where staff don't hide behind their titles and pretend to understand what they don't yet understand.

A humane mental health service is one where people are treated with dignity and pain is respected as a form of intelligence. Services where symptoms are viewed as survival strategies and stories are evolved with service users that 'fit the landscape of their experience' and include the social context of a person's life.

There are many options for doing this. Psychologists use 'formulations' to connect a person's presenting difficulties with key events in their childhood, their vulnerabilities and strengths, current threats and triggers in their lives, and how all of these relate to the particular way in which that person experiences distress.

A very promising alternative to psychiatric classification – which I am currently using in my work with the homeless – is the Power Threat Meaning Framework (PTMF). Developed by Lucy Johnstone and Mary Boyle under the auspices of the British Psychological Society, the PTMF is a radical approach to understanding emotional distress and restoring hope. It is a series of intriguing questions that co-create with someone the story of their lives. People's strengths and difficulties are explored but not through the lens of individual psychiatric diagnoses or psychological deficits. Instead, the PTMF focuses on the role of power imbalances in their lives, the impact of the resulting threats, how they make sense of their experiences, and the strategies they used and still use to survive. We can all use this model to craft a 'story' of why we feel and behave as we do.

As mental health professionals, we are the instruments of our work. We learn primarily by experience, coupled with reflection and supervision. A humane mental health service is one where staff are encouraged and supported to reflect formally on their interactions. It is unforgivable for us not to be aware of what we are doing and how we are doing it with extremely sensitive people. It is not *treatments,* but how we *treat* people that determines the outcome.

Every professional in the mental health field needs to be trained in person-centred listening and how to build and maintain relationships with service users and their families. We need clinicians, including psychiatrists, to train in various forms of therapy appropriate to their skills and interest. Staff will need good supervision from seasoned in-house psychotherapists. We need to be able to offer a range of therapeutic interventions, including those which speak to difficult problems. Deeper forms of therapy and comprehensive multidisciplinary teamwork will be required for people with severe and enduring mental health vulnerabilities. We need a range of therapeutic skills in services rather than a single brand of psychotherapy.

If it takes a village to raise a child, it takes a community to enable people to face severe mental health difficulties. Our services should be an integral part of the community. Close collaboration with service user organisations and movements can teach us about recovery. We can improve our programmes by incorporating their hard-won wisdom.

We have to reform our public mental health campaigns. People need to know that most mental health difficulties arise from early childhood experiences or social circumstances that are oppressive and unjust.

Finally, we need to evolve mental health services that are healing to people, families and communities but also speak more broadly and loudly to our society about how we are driving each other 'mad' through some of the conditions, expectations and social aspirations we accept as 'normal'. Most of what we call 'mental illness' is caused by interpersonal experiences and social circumstances. Yet, as mental health professionals, we have surprisingly little to say about how certain cultural practices and social inequalities impact our well-being. It is not enough just to give useful 'tips' about how to cope with emotional difficulties; we must challenge how we create those difficulties in the first place.

THE HEART'S CALLING

t was strange to find myself stepping onto the St Patrick's Cathedral pulpit to deliver the only sermon I would ever give. I was a Christian Brothers boy, raised Catholic, and not a member of any religious institution. Yet here I was, midway through a Protestant High Mass, about to speak to a formidable audience, including our Taoiseach and over a thousand secondary school students. Even as I climbed those steps, I wasn't sure what I would say.

In 2016, the Board of the Church of Ireland Secondary Schools decided to make mental health the theme of the coming academic year for their 22 schools all over Ireland. To bless this endeavour, students from each school were invited to St Patrick's Cathedral for a special ceremony. A convoy of buses decanted them at the cathedral gates. Uniformed teenagers piled out and entered the iconic building. They squeezed into every available pew and filled rows of added chairs that lined the aisles and the spacious area at the back of the cathedral.

Because of my work with young people, I had been invited by the Dean to speak to these students about their mental health. Before the liturgy began, I was shown a particular ornate wooden chair in the choir stalls with the designation 'Prebendary of Newcastle' over it. When I had met a week earlier with the Dean to be briefed for the event, he had told me with a wry smile that for that one day, I would assume the role of prebendary since it was a custom of the cathedral that only people who held a formal office could deliver a sermon. I learned that a 'prebendary' was a canon of the cathedral whose income (or 'prebend') came from a particular township.

Alone on the throne, I listened to the choir as their singing mixed with rising incense and the quiet hum of a packed church. When it was time, the verger came to where I was sitting, bowed and beckoned me to follow him to the pulpit. I looked at the white marble architecture and thought of Johnathan Swift, who must have climbed these steps many times. I stepped into a circular speaking area richly lined with red velvet. I looked out on the sea of fresh-faced teenagers in school uniforms and familiar-looking dignitaries in the front rows. I addressed everyone appropriately. And then, after a pause, I said: 'You are facing a new year. I can say with certainty that two things will happen to each of you in the year ahead: You will have good times, and you will have bad times. I'm assuming you can all probably handle the good times. I'm here to talk about the bad times.'

By that stage, I knew something about 'bad' times. They happen to all of us, often when we least expect them. Some painful experience erupts, leaving us disoriented and unsure of what to do next.

I've had the privilege of meeting people who have had more than their share of painful moments. They bore the scars of very difficult lives. Many had carried their wounds with dignity until they had reached a breaking point where they could no longer do so. Their vulnerability created a unique opportunity for honest conversations that didn't routinely happen in the 'normal' world. Some had become embittered by their pain, which seemed impossible to resolve or escape. But most struggled to find themselves and make sense of their lives.

They accepted support, despite believing for years that they would have to go it alone. Together we faced their fear and bewilderment, sadness and rage. We allowed what had been disowned room to breathe. In time, their fragmented emotions and memories began to tell a more coherent story. While it may have been terrifying, their distress often revealed an inner strength they had never known they had.

It usually takes longer than the books appreciate to recover a sense of Self. Recovery can be tedious. Healing is usually a work in progress rather than a brief journey with a happy ending. Despite its challenges and setbacks, recovery always brings people closer to their humanity. Which in turn gives people like me, who are part of that journey, an opportunity to deepen our own.

What I told those students in the cathedral was something I had learned from working with people at the edge. When we can face what is difficult in our lives, however painful that may be, however long that may take, we grow; but when we deny, avoid or repress what hurts, we can become stuck in our lives.

Inevitably there will be times when we all feel 'bad'. It can be hard to acknowledge this, and we may try to push it away. Sometimes, the best we can do to cope with a distressing experience is to push it away. In the immediate aftermath of a shock, we instinctively block it out because it is too hard to take in. While our defensive behaviours may help in the short term, they can backfire in the long term. We always learn something important if we can take a moment to be with what feels 'uncomfortable' and what doesn't feel right. When we can listen, rather than push it away, it points us to something, or someone, that needs our attention and care. Emotional pain is a form of intelligence. It deserves our respect.

I reminded these students that mental health is not about 'feeling good' or 'feeling bad'; mental health is about being connected with reality and with each other. It is about knowing how I am doing on any given day and asking myself: 'What do I need?' 'What might help?' 'How much of this problem can I deal with now, and what do I leave for another time?'

Facing reality is probably the most difficult thing for human beings, especially when it's hard. As a species, we seem hell-bent on forgetting our troubles. Society bombards us daily with an infinite number of ways to distract ourselves. We are constantly reminded to be 'positive'. Easy solutions and quick fixes are offered to complex challenges in our lives. Reflection is discouraged as we rush headlong into a future where we are promised that a better life awaits us.

Feeling good is delightful and should be enjoyed for the gift it is. But, for this congregation of students, taking care of their mental health would involve keeping their wits about them. The world they were stepping into was complicated. It held many wonders and opportunities for them to explore. But it could also kill them as quickly as it looked at them. They would need to learn to listen to themselves. And to trust that whatever they were feeling, there would always be a very good reason why they felt that way.

Finally, I told them that nobody makes it on their own. The human species is not equipped with exceptional talents to survive. We don't have a lion's strength or a gazelle's speed. We are immensely vulnerable. Our bodies are unguarded and open to the world. We may dream of having some superpower, but we never will. Our secret to survival lies in our capacity to form and sustain relationships with one another. We need people in our lives who trust and believe in us. Reaching out to them for support is not a sign of weakness. It is a sign of strength. In doing so, we are being true to our deeper nature.

Writing this book has meant a lot to me. If it has a message, it would be to open your heart, learn from the experiences and people that life puts in your way, and be passionate about whatever you do.

My journey of recovery is not at an end yet. It will likely never be. But something has changed. I'm more aware of what can upend me. I've accepted that I find some situations very hurtful. Rather than fight with my reactions, I accept them. I feel what I feel. Rather than push painful emotions away, I allow them to run their course and give myself time to recover. And if I need support, I'm not ashamed to ask for it. My life has been a search to find a secure base in myself. Security isn't achieved through any one single person or experience, but through being open and responsive to different opportunities life gives us along the way.

In 2012, Ursula and I traded our house in Dublin for a bungalow on the edge of a cliff in Sligo. We did it up. We planted over 1,000 shrubs and trees, created several large vegetable and herb beds and populated the garden with animals.

Maybe it's the sea, its rocky shores, its windswept grasses; maybe it's the company of animals or the kindness of a small group of neighbours who respect boundaries but are really generous to a fault; but on this headland at the heart of Yeats Country, with its fierce salt-water gales and soft blue light that wraps itself around Benbulbin, I have found the stranger who was myself.

I have found security through learning to value practical, everyday activities. Having built an identity around being spontaneous, open and always ready to seize new opportunities, I now appreciate the simple routines I previously dismissed. A child's security depends on being loved in a consistent, reliable way. Our adult Self also needs consistency and some level of predictability. Having a rhythm in our day where we pay attention to simple chores and responsibilities grounds us.

My day starts with taking heart medication, brushing my teeth, emptying the dishwasher, feeding chickens, rabbits, cats and wild birds, and making porridge and coffee. Ideally, I circle the headland and complete a simple exercise routine. I am more consistent than before in my meditation practice. I honour these daily routines not because I 'should' but because they give a rhythm to the day that steadies me.

My imagination remains my inner shed. Since discovering mindfulness, I've been able to revamp it completely and repurpose it. It is much more spacious and user-friendly. Some days my shed is where I sink into the sheer joy of simply being alive; some days, I go there when I'm overly tired, worked up about a difficult conversation, or stressed by responsibilities and deadlines. And while it can be a place of escape, it can also be a place where I can face difficulties rather than avoid them.

One irony of my lifestyle here is that I spend much of my time behind glass. When we added an extension to the side of the house, we dug down into the ground and made it two storeys. The gable end is made entirely of glass. Wall-to-wall, ceiling-to-floor. The main bedroom is upstairs, my study is downstairs. I think it ironic that my troubles started as a child behind a glassed-in crib, where I spent four weeks. My life has come full circle to where I find myself, once again, behind glass. Of course, it is different. As an infant of two years old, I was trapped, cut off from everyone and everything familiar to me. Now I look through this glass at a landscape to which I feel deeply connected. Life has welcomed me to this place and given me a home.

The parts of me that were disowned for so long have a place at the table. We have learned to appreciate each other's company. Our conversations are always interesting.

Life changes when we have adult children and grandchildren. There are surprises every week. Someone has just crossed a milestone and astounded their parents. Someone is homesick or singing in public for the first time. With modern technology, the time interval between these giant steps is measured in nanoseconds. News, complete with visual aids, arrives in real time.

My passion has been for mental health and how we care for those whose hearts have been broken. Since I started my work in 1976, I have witnessed people have a range of experiences at the hands of our services—some good, some not at all good. I think that now, we are in crisis. Mainly because we have over-medicalised human suffering by reducing the meaning of our pain to diseases rather than to relationship experiences, history and social circumstances.

If my concerns have been mostly targeted at psychiatry, it is because they hold a completely disproportionate level of power in the mental health system. The justification for their power is their claim that mental and emotional pain is an illness rather than the legacy of what happened and may still be happening to people in their lives. As doctors, they offer a unique contribution, but as carers of the human heart, they are often ill-equipped.

I went along with this way of thinking for years until I worked with young people and saw how they are being medicalised more and more. I am concerned that early intervention – which I heartily support – may also draw people into unnecessary long-term psychiatric care. Once labelled and assigned a medication regime, children and young people are primed to be referred to adult services. Should they hit any existential crisis in their lives, they and their families are likely to consider it a reoccurrence of their 'mental illness'. Even the most ethical psychiatrist may be tempted to extend their drug regime indefinitely. After all, they will argue, better to be safe than sorry.

My anger is with any form of superficial, lazy or conceited approach to service users, whatever profession is involved. I am concerned about children and adults entrusted to their care who may buy into all they are told. People in an emotional crisis are in such a vulnerable place. Their future sense of identity, how they relate to their inner world, make sense of their pain and how others see them can depend on the wisdom of their doctor. Many of the problems we currently have in the mental health service are not due to a chemical imbalance but to a power imbalance.

Service users are becoming more vocal and are speaking out for themselves. This deserves all our support. Some people are writing the story of their career as psychiatric patients, and their accounts will be as shocking as they are common. But I'm aware that many service users will not speak out. They fear being 'punished' in subtle ways if they do. Being told that they 'lack insight' if they disagree with the doctor. They may have their meds increased, be placed in a more 'secure' ward, have their phones removed, or find it harder to get an appointment should they ask for one.

I don't write just to complain. I write because I know we have the insights and tools to do a lot better. Resources are a major issue but we also need to rethink our paradigm of the way we offer care to address deep psychosocial needs. People also need therapeutic, family and social care in addition to medical care. I would like every profession to have basic therapeutic skills and to commit to some forum where staff collectively reflect on these skills. Our aim should be to make our mental health centres places where there is a safe, contained therapeutic milieu.

Somewhere in the mix, we need to see the presence of 'experts-by-experience', people who have been shattered but survived and found themselves through all of it. Their empathy can reach further and deeper than ours. Inviting them to be part of our teams will help us all to be more honest about how effective our services are.

Story plays a powerful role in our lives. When we can

transform 'the memory of our suffering into an acceptable work of art', as Freud wrote, 'we are no longer victims of it'. Our stories can be both a comfort and a caution to others. They can reveal different possibilities that pain opens for all of us. Our services need a bigger story, a more hopeful paradigm for how to think about, talk about and respond to the mental health needs of this country. Our young people particularly need stories that inspire them. A mythology that maps their path and tells them what to expect.

Our family grew up watching the PBS production *The Power of Myth* featuring the mythologist Joseph Campbell. That series of six programmes laid out what he called The Hero's Journey. It was before my daughter Rachel's time, but the boys loved it, and it has served them well.

The hero's journey is the journey we are all called to make. Our personal path is where we discover who we are and make something of our lives. Life constantly invites us to undertake a challenge, let go and embrace some change in our circumstances. Fear is our natural response to the unknown and the unfamiliar. The essence of a heroic journey is that we face whatever we fear.

We may say 'no' as often as we say 'yes' to the call to adventure. But the desire to grow is something we can never completely silence. It's that small voice in the quiet of our hearts that prompts us to do something with our lives. What it promises in return for our 'yes' is a path in life where we will embody our truth and speak with our voice.

Where that path leads us is unpredictable. We will get hurt because every hero is wounded in some way; we may experience a profound letting go of some part of our familiar selves that feels like death because, in every heroic quest, someone or something dies. The journey may be a messy affair, one that takes us through places of confusion and darkness.

We must be attentive and open to the support that life offers us along the way. The heroes of all time have been graced with 'spirit guides' to show them their way in and out of the labyrinth. These guides may be our teachers, our therapists, through whom we learn the key skills to survive and complete our journey. They can be firm with us and expose our tendencies to read things incorrectly and bring about our own downfall. They show us how tiny adjustments in our navigation can bring us through troubled waters. They may teach us to accept what is broken in us and hold it with compassion, viewing it not as an obstacle but as something that gives us a unique way of seeing in the dark. Our most powerful guide is our awareness of where we are at any moment.

In every myth, legend and fairy tale, there comes a moment when the hero must confront some demon. We all have to face our demons at some point, but they are not born of some evil within us. They are the expression of our fear. They may appear as voices within that try to persuade us that what we seek, our heart's calling, is something we will never achieve, something we do not deserve. Sometimes we defeat our demons; mostly, we tame them and harness their intelligence to help us achieve our quest.

When we have faced our demons, we are ready to enter what Campbell called 'the land of miracles'. Here we see our lives afresh, experience the vitality of being alive and feel connected with all living things – most importantly, ourselves. This is an experience of bliss. It is tempting to want to put down roots in this place and stay here forever. But while our journey has taken us inwards to this place, its purpose has always been to discover some truth we can share with others. The final part of the hero's journey is the return to one's community with some treasure – a gem of wisdom.

Myths express universal truths. These stories alert us to the dark energies in human beings that can cripple us, deceive us and seduce us. The function of myth is to communicate that there is also the capacity to find our way in each of us. And that there is within the universe an intrinsic goodness that will support us as we respond to the call to become human.

Joseph Campbell's gift was to discern a healing order underlying apparent chaos, to reveal beauty at the heart of darkness. He once said, 'You are the mystery you seek to know'. Awakening to that mystery and discovering how deeply interconnected we are with each other is the journey of the human heart.

And we don't have to risk this adventure alone,

for the heroes of all time have gone before us.
The labyrinth is thoroughly known ...
we have only to follow the thread of the hero path ...

And where we had thought to slay another
we shall slay ourselves.
Where we had thought to travel outwards
we shall come to the centre of our own existence.
And where we had thought to be alone
we shall be with all the world.[1]

EPILOGUE

WHAT I'VE LEARNED ABOUT PAIN

In the most painful corners of our experience, something alive is always waiting to emerge. So whatever pain or problem we have, if it helps us find a quality of presence – where we can open to it, see it, feel it, include it, and find the truth concealed in it – that is our healing.[1]

JOHN WELWOOD

At the end of this book, I'm thinking about what writing this book has meant to me and what I hope it might mean to you. We've both had our struggles. You know more about mine than I may ever know about yours. From an early age I've had questions that have been like an itch I had to scratch. They were born out of loss in my childhood, gained momentum through a turbulent adolescence and became inescapable in adulthood when I saw what was unresolved in me hurt the people I cared about. How can we come to terms with traumas in our lives and not be broken by them? Can our pain make us more rather than less human? This book is my attempt to answer these questions. Many people have helped me, psychology has so often lit the way for me and my work with people who confronted their own personal demons has always inspired me to keep going. Like Campbell's hero, I've walked my own path and confronted ordeals.

Pain has been an important teacher in my life. It had broken my heart when I didn't want it to. I thought I was happy living alone inside my head for years, but I was half-living in a safe hell. I needed to have the protective layer around my heart broken open to taste what life was really about.

How do you relate to pain when it drops into your life? When some loss or a setback pulls the rug of security out from under you, are you as frightened of it as I was? Do you resent it? Do you go to great lengths not to feel how vulnerable you are?

Emotional pain can be a lonely, exhausting and frightening experience. While the rest of the world is fine and getting on with their lives, you're stuck in a place where all you can think about is the effort it takes to walk from one end of the house to the other.

You face each day with good intentions. You make a list of things you need to do. You try to keep it realistic, given how little energy you have. But even the simplest list can feel too much. Pain slows all of us to a crawl.

You worry that something is wrong with you as a person. Surely 'normal' people never feel this bad? We live in a world where there seems to be no place for emotional suffering. The bandwidth of feelings we tolerate as a society has become very narrow. Hurting people are viewed as overly sensitive and unable to keep up with the crowd. Although people may not say it explicitly, they silently wonder why we don't pull ourselves together and move on with our lives. They don't realise that we ask ourselves those same questions every day.

There are a few things that I have found helpful in such moments. Above all, I need someone who recognises that my pain is real. It makes an enormous difference when someone 'gets' how badly I feel. I don't need them to take away my pain but to let me know it's okay to feel it. And to trust that there is a good reason why I feel the way I do, even when I can't see what that is.

Pain always means something. My hurt, anxiety, low mood and frustrations are messengers. They point me to what needs my attention. Perhaps some old wound has re-opened and needs more care. Where I live, or work, may be more stressful than I realise. Maybe someone said something that upset me more than I felt it should. I can beat myself up for letting life get to me, or I can accept that sometimes that's exactly what it does.

When pain is intense, I feel trapped inside it. For a while, all I can see is pain. I can't think clearly. Frightening thoughts and feelings swirl around inside my mind. I feel myself slipping down an all-too-familiar rabbit hole and can't seem to control my fall.

Later, I can step back a little when my emotions have settled. I can see that I am hurting. With that awareness comes some compassion. I wouldn't wish this on anyone. I stop fighting with myself. I try to allow myself to be exactly how I already am.

Mindfulness has helped. It has given me a different, kinder way to relate to my experience. But it has taken lots of practice. I check in with my body and notice my internal 'weather'. I find some way to anchor myself in the present. This can be the rhythm of my in-breath and out-breath or the contact between my body and whatever supports me. And when I'm grounded, mindfulness invites me to move towards my pain rather than away from it. If I am sad, I accept that I am sad and allow myself to be sad. I can stay a while with my feelings and listen to what they may be trying to say to me. I may be angry, but being aware of my anger makes it less likely that I will express it harmfully. I explore the raw edges of my experience with curiosity and kindness.

When we contract against our pain, we intensify it. When we ignore or repress unwanted feelings, they fester and linger on. Disowned hurt and anger seep through as anxiety, tension, worry or persistent insecurity. Denying our grief and sadness can leave us lacking energy, interest and motivation.

But what if our pain is more than we can manage? In that case, it may be enough to acknowledge that a particular situation or stress is very upsetting and leave it at that. To give ourselves a break from strong emotions with a promise to return to them. Recognising our distress and reminding ourselves that we're doing our best to survive may be enough.

Deep wounds need time to heal. This book is proof of that

in my own life. I've had to feel the hurt I carried for years many times over. This has been exhausting at times. It's hard to visit and revisit memories and emotions I imagined I'd already come to terms with. But I've noticed that each time I do, even briefly, the wounds of my past heal a little more.

Pain has taught me to ask myself what might help. Sometimes the best and the wisest thing I can do is to lie down and allow my pain to settle. On other occasions, I need to walk or talk to a trusted friend. When you ask yourself what you need or what might help, you will find your answers.

Being able to connect in a genuine, open-hearted way with another person is always healing. Sometimes that person may also be hurting. As a psychologist, I stepped into the world of deeply sensitive people who had struggled emotionally more than I ever had and found permission to be human. I found hope in the openness and vulnerability of people I thought I was meant to 'fix'. There were boundaries that we observed and confidences that we each respected. But above all, when trust grew between us, we both experienced an intense dose of human contact that was life-giving.

The time will come when you and I will be asked to be there for someone else in pain. This can be hard, particularly when that person is someone we care about. We would do anything to ease their pain. It is tempting to offer explanations, advice or solutions to make things easier for them. While these may help, the risk is that we take them away from their pain and allow them to fall back into their familiar identity.

They may welcome a break from their distress, but ultimately, everything stays the same.

When Freud reflected on his work as a therapist late in his life, he realised that it wasn't enough for people to have their pain explained to them; to heal, they needed to experience it. Our presence and our listening can make it safe for others to feel what they feel. And at the raw edges of their pain, they may find a truth that changes their life.

I hope you are less frightened of having your heart broken open after reading this book. Because when it happens, as it inevitably will, you have a chance to become more human. To discover a tenderness in yourself that you didn't know you could feel. To realise in a whole new way how fragile and how amazing you are.

ACKNOWLEDGEMENTS

Thanks to Sarah Liddy, Margaret Farrelly and the team at Gill for the care they took of this story from its inception. Thanks also to my gifted editor, Kerri Ward, for making my life readable and our work together so invigorating. And to Michael Gill for building such a unique publishing company.

To Helen Shaw, who suggested the title and reminded me that universal truths are more credible when grounded in personal experience. To Micheline Egan, who has helped me to find my voice as a writer over many years and has been involved with this project every step of the way. Deep gratitude to Michael Sanderson, Gwen Hempenstall, Mia Gallagher, Simon Sleeman, Bob Illback and Brian Leyden, who read sections of this book as it evolved and gave me invaluable feedback. And to Marian McGorrin, whose insights helped me to bring the final draft over the finish line.

To those who shaped and formed the psychologist I've become, including Therese Brady, Helen Haughton, John Dunne, Des Hourihane, Ann Murphy, Gillian Butler, Eamonn Butler, Brendan Murphy, Mark Williams, Dom Michael Ryan, Julie Kinchla, Annie Rogers, Lucy Johnstone, Brenda

Doherty, Eamonn Gaffney, Tim Beck, David Burns, Jeremy Holmes and Barbara Dooley.

My thanks to Marian Finucane and Anne Farrell in RTÉ and Kevin O'Sullivan in the *Irish Times*. You opened doors that changed my career. Thank you to Frank Kelly, Deirdre McHugh, Breda O'Toole, Clive Shannon, Catherine Redmond and the Coyle family, who shared their journey and kept me honest.

Thanks to Rosaleen McElvaney, who believed I had a book in me long before I did. To Liagh Miller and the Bellevue Book Club, who broadened my literary horizons and stretched my imagination. And to Eamon Mag Uidhir, my first writing mentor.

I am critical of psychiatry in this book for how it can over-medicalise emotional distress, obscure the psychological and social roots of our pain and misuse its power in relating to people in a very vulnerable place in their lives. But I am also mindful of former colleagues in psychiatry whose humanity and care of their patients were exemplary. I'm thinking especially of Michael Gill, Marcus Webb, Brian Lawlor, Brian Fitzmaurice, Karen O'Connor, Declan Lyons, Pat Bracken, Ivor Browne, George Mullett and Anthony Clare. I especially thank my colleagues in St James's Hospital, including occupational therapist Vicky Love and community nurses Eamonn Kelly and Michael O'Driscoll, who always saw dignity in the people they cared for.

Thank you to friends and neighbours whose encouragement and support have meant more than they can ever know: James McGrath, who looked after the animals and my garden while I was immersed in this project. The Smith family: Lorraine, Rachael, Shauna and Aela-Rae, whose care for each other inspired me. Thanks to Jackie and Brendan Marren, Bernie and Teresa Murray, Emer Duggan, Maria Melody, Andie Kenny, Mary McDonnell, Kevin Doherty, Barbara and Ted Kelly, Denise and Bill Whelan, and Paula Naughton for their warmth and support. My thanks to my neighbours on this headland who have shown me what real community is about. To Martin at RTÉ Sligo for his kindness throughout Covid.

Thanks also to Kevin O'Higgins, Marianne Lipson, Brid Grant, Michael Lally, Aideen Loftus, Dhara Kelly, Seamus O'Donnell, Louize Carroll and Niall Breslin, whose friendship has been so important in my life. John O'Leary and the band of brothers I lived with during college meant the world to me. My gratitude to the team at Jigsaw, past and present, especially the young people who taught me so much about vulnerability and resilience. To Declan Ryan, whose generosity and concern for young people made Jigsaw possible.

Thanks to Sr Stan, Sr Sile, Jane Negrych, Brother Richard Hendrik, Gary Graham, Barry Lee and the team in the Sanctuary, who've always nourished my heart. To doctors John Latham and Ted Keelan, who kept my actual heart beating.

A deep bow to Ciara Carty and the many people I've come to know through my work with Focus Ireland. Your commitment to creating homes for people who don't feel they belong anywhere has been a privilege to witness. Your compassion and consistency have shown me that psychological healing is possible even in the darkest corners of human suffering.

Love to my siblings: Kevin, Mel and Miriam, who shared our family's wonders and idiosyncrasies.

To Ursula for the journey we've shared through thick and thin, and to our children and grandchildren Luca, Alanna, Noah, Zoe and Isla.

REFERENCES

Introduction

1 Rachel Aviv. *Strangers to Ourselves: Unsettled Minds and the Stories That Make Us.* New York: Farrar, Straus and Giroux, 2022. p.22.

Chapter One

1 Edith Eger. *The Choice: Embrace the Possible.* London: Rider, 2018.
2 Boris Cyrulnik. *Resilience.* London: Penguin, 2009. 10-11.
3 Bruce Perry and Oprah Winfrey. *What Happened To You? Conversations on Trauma, Resilience and Healing.* London: Pan Macmillan, 2021. 58-59.

Chapter Two

1 Annie Rogers. Public talk given in Dublin, Ireland, 2012.

Chapter Three

1 W.R. Bion. *Attention and Interpretation.* Oxfordshire: Routledge, 1970. 42.
2 John Bowlby. *A Secure Base: Clinical Applications of Attachment Theory.* Oxfordshire: Routledge, 1988.
3 James Robertson. *A 2-year-old Goes to Hospital.* Robertson Films, 1952. http://www.concordmedia.org.uk/products/a-two-year-old-goes-to-hospital-52/
4 James and Joyce Robertson. *Separation and the Very Young.* London: Free Association Books, 1989. 97 and 140.

5 J.D. Matarazzo. 'David Wechsler (1896-1981)'. *American Psychologist*, 36. 12 (1981): 1542–1543.

6 Theodora Alcock. *The Rorschach in Practice*. Philadelphia: J.B Lippincott, 1963.

7 Arron Beck. *Cognitive Therapy of Depression*. New York: Guilford Press, 1979.

8 Robbie Case 'Piaget's theory of child development and its implications'. *Phi Delta Kappan*, 55. 1 (1973).

9 Jeremy Holmes, 'Raj Persaud chats to Jeremy Holmes', YouTube, 2017. https://www.youtube.com/watch?v=UHTuYRE6I4o

10 David Smail, *Illusion and Reality: The Meaning of Anxiety*. London: J.M. Dent and Sons, 1984. 141.

Chapter Five

1 Alice Miller, *The Body Never Lies: The Lingering Effects of Hurtful Parenting*. New York: W. W. Norton & Company, 2006.

Chapter Six

1 William Butler Yeats. *The Collected Poems of W.B. Yeats*. London: Palgrave Macmillan, 1991.

Chapter Seven

1 Derek Scally, *The Best Catholics in the World: The Irish, the Church and the End of a Special Relationship*. London: Penguin, 2022.

2 Geraldine Moane, *Gender and Colonialism: A Psychological Analysis of Oppression and Liberation*. London: Palgrave Macmillan, 2010.

3 Wilfred Bion. *Learning from Experience*. New York: Jason Aronson, 1983. 72.

Chapter Eight

1   Mark Aveline, *From Medicine to Psychotherapy*. London: Whurr Publishers, 1992. 4.

2   Nina Coltart. *Slouching towards Bethlehem*. Manila: Phoenix Publishing House, 2021. 118.

3   D.W. Winnicott. *Playing and Reality*. New York: New York Basic Books, 1971. 57. Quoted in Marilyn Charles, *Learning from Experience: A Guidebook for Clinicians*. London: Routledge, 2004.

4   Michael Balint. *The Basic Fault: Therapeutic Aspects of Regression*. Northwestern University Press, 1992.

5   Hal and Sidra Stone. *Embracing Ourselves: The Voice Dialogue Manual*. New Delhi: Nataraj Publishing, 1998.

6   Bessel van der Kolk. *The Body Keeps the Score: Mind, Brain and Body in the Transformation of Trauma*. London: Penguin, 2014. 97.

7   Michael Visceglia / Suzanne Vega. 'Language', BMG Rights Management, Warner Chappell Music, Inc, 1987.

8   Marilyn Charles, *Learning from Experience: A Guidebook for Clinicians*. London: Routledge, 2004. 108.

Chapter Nine

1   Alice Miller, *The Body Never Lies: The Lingering Effects of Hurtful Parenting*. New York: W. W. Norton & Company, 2006.

2   Wilfred Bion. *Learning from Experience*. New York: Jason Aronson, 1983. 72.

Chapter Ten

1   Marilyn Charles and Michael O'Loughlin (2012) 'The complex subject of psychosis'. *Psychoanalysis, Culture & Society*, 17 (2012): 418. doi:10.1057/pcs.2012.3.

2   Jon Kabat-Zinn. *Full Catastrophe Living*. London: Random House, 1990. 168.

3   Rachel Aviv. *Strangers to Ourselves: Unsettled Minds and the Stories That Make Us.* New York: Farrar, Straus and Giroux, 2022. 22 and 24.

Chapter Eleven

1   Emily Dickinson. *The Complete Poems.* London: Faber and Faber, 2016.
2   Darian Leader. *What is Madness?* London: Penguin, 2011. 96.
3   Richard Ellman. *James Joyce.* North Carolina: Oxford University Press USA, 1984.
4   J. Read, J. van Os, A. Morrison and C. Ross. 'Childhood trauma, psychosis and schizophrenia: A literature review with theoretical and clinical implications.' *Acta Psychiatrica Scandanavica,* 112. 5 (2005): 330–350.
5   M. Birchwood, A. Meaden, P. Trower, P. Gilbert, J. Plaistow. 'The power and omnipotence of voices: subordination and entrapment by voices and significant others.' *Psychological Medicine,* 30. 2 (1994): 337-44. Also, Dan Olweus. 'Bullying at School: Basic Facts and Effects of a School Based Intervention Program.' *Journal of Child Psychology and Psychiatry,* 35. 7 (1994): 1171-1190.
6   I. Kelleher, D Connor, M.C. Clarke, N Devlin, M Harley, M Cannon. 'Prevalence of psychotic symptoms in childhood and adolescence: a systematic review and meta-analysis of population-based studies.' *Psychological Medicine,* 9 (2012): 1-7.
7   Elyn Saks. *The Centre Cannot Hold: My Journey through Madness.* New York: Hyperion, 2007. 168. Quoted by Annie Rogers in *Incandescent Alphabets: Psychosis and the Enigma of Language.* London: Karnac, 2016.
8   Robert Whitaker. *Anatomy of an Epidemic: Magic Bullets, Psychiatric Drugs, and the Astonishing Rise of Mental Illness in America.* London: Crown, 2010.
9   B.C. Ho, N. Andreasen and S. Ziebell. (2011) 'Long-term

antipsychotic treatment and brain volumes: a longitudinal study of first-episode schizophrenia.' *Archives of General Psychiatry.* 68. 2 (2011): 128-137.

10 G. Chouinard, B. Jones. 'Schizophrenia as dopamine-deficiency disease.' Lancet, 8.2 (1978): 99-100.

11 M. Harrow, T.H. Jobe. 'Does long-term treatment of schizophrenia with antipsychotic medications facilitate recovery?' *Schizophrenia Bulletin*, 39. 5 (2013): 962-965. doi: 10.1093/schbul/sbt034. Epub 19 March 2013.

12 J. Seikkula, B. Alakare and J. Aaltonen. 'The comprehensive open-dialogue approach (II). Long-term stability of acute psychosis outcomes in advanced community care: The Western Lapland Project.' *ResearchGate*, 2011.

13 'The 388, A Psychoanalytic Center for the Treatment of Psychosis', www.madinamerica.com/provider-directory/150222/388-psychoanalytic-center-treatment-psychosis.

14 Gary Donohoe and Karen O'Connor, 'Early intervention in psychosis.' In *Understanding Youth Mental Health: Perspectives From Theory and Practice*, eds E. Hennessy., C. Heary and M. Michail. Open University Press, 2022. 149-165.

15 Annie Rogers. *Incandescent Alphabets: Psychosis and the Enigma of Language*. London: Karnac, 2016. 151.

16 Darian Leader. *What is Madness?* London: Penguin, 2011. 294.

17 Annie Rogers. *Incandescent Alphabets: Psychosis and the Enigma of Language*. London: Karnac, 2016. 151.

18 Darian Leader. *What is Madness?* London: Penguin, 2011. 296.

19 Tony Bates. *One of the Family*. Dublin: Health Education Bureau, 1981.

20 Quoted in Nina Coltart, *Slouching towards Bethlehem*. Manila: Phoenix Publishing House, 2021. 194.

Chapter Twelve

1 Nikita Gill. *These are the Words: Fearless Verse to Find your Voice*. New York: Macmillan, 2022.

2   Marilyn Charles, *Learning from Experience: A Guidebook for Clinicians*. London: Routledge, 2004. 31-32.

3   John Welwood. *Toward a Psychology of Awakening*. Colorado: Shambhala Publications, 2002. 173.

4   Carl Jung. *Memories, Dreams, Reflections*. New York: Pantheon Books, 1963. 191.

5   Anthony Storr. *Jung*. New York: Routledge, 1991. 83.

6   Anthony Storr. *Feet of Clay*. New York: Harper Collins, 1997. 92.

7   NHS Business Services Authority. 'Medicines used in Mental Health 2015/16 – 2021/22.'

8   Kirsten Shukla, *The Pharmaceutical Journal*, 307. 7953 (2021).

9   Northwestern University. 'Why antidepressants don't work for so many.' ScienceDaily, 27 Oct 2009. www.sciencedaily.com/releases/2009/10/091023163346.htm.

10 J. Glenmullen. *Prozac Backlash: Overcoming the Dangers of Prozac, Zoloft, Paxil and Other Antidepressants with Safe, Effective Alternatives*. New York: Simon and Schuster, 2001. 384.

11 Steven H. Aggen, Michael C. Neale and Kenneth S. Kendler. 'DSM criteria for major depression: evaluating symptom patterns using latent-trait item response models.' *Psychological Medicine*, 35 (2005): 475–487.

12 J. Moncrieff, R.E. Cooper, T. Stockmann, et al. 'The serotonin theory of depression: a systematic umbrella review of the evidence.' *Mol Psychiatry* (2022): https://doi.org/10.1038/s41380-022-01661.

13 American Psychiatric Association. 'What is depression?' https://www.psychiatry.org/patients-families/depression/what-is-depression.

14 Nikita Gill. *These are the Words: Fearless Verse to Find your Voice*. New York: Macmillan, 2022.

Chapter Thirteen

1   B. Illback, T. Bates and C. Hodges, C. et al. 'Jigsaw: Engaging communities in the development and implementation of youth

mental health services and supports in the Republic of Ireland.' *Journal of Mental Health*, 19.5 (2010): 422–435.

2   B. Dooley, and A. Fitzgerald. 'My World Survey: National Study of Youth Mental Health in Ireland', 2012: http://www.ucd.ie/t4cms/MyWorldSurvey.pdf.

3   Mark Katz. *On Playing a Poor Hand Well*. New York: W.W. Norton & Company, 1997.

4   Sami Timimi. *A Straight Talking Introduction to Children's Mental Health Problems* (2nd edition), PCCS Books , 2020. 38.

Chapter Fourteen

1   L. Johnstone. *A Straight Talking Introduction to Psychiatric Diagnosis*, revised second edition. PCCS Books, 2022.

2   M.C. Angermeyer, A. Holzinger, M.G. Carta, G. Schomerus, *Biogenetic explanations and public acceptance of mental illness: systematic review of population studies*. The British Journal of Psychiatry, 199 (2011): 367–72.

3   J. Read, N. Haslam and L. Magliano. 'Prejudice, stigma and 'schizophrenia': The role of bio-genetic ideology.' In *Models of Madness: Psychological, Social and Biological Approaches to Psychosis*. Eds J. Read and J. Dillon. London: Routledge, 2013. 191-209.

4   T. Moses. 'Self-labelling and its effects among adolescents diagnosed with mental disorders.' *Social Science and Medicine*, 68. 3 (2009): 570-578.

5   A. Frances. 'Saving Normal. An insider's revolt against out-of-control psychiatric diagnosis, DSM-5, big pharma and the medicalisation of ordinary life.' *Psychotherapy in Australia*, 19. 3 (2013): 14-18. Quoted in L. Johnstone, *A Straight Talking Introduction to Psychiatric Diagnosis*. Wales: PCCS Books, 2022.

6   Office of the High Commissioner for Human Rights. *Special Rapporteur on the right to physical and mental health*. Office of the High Commissioner for Human Rights, 2017.

7 Shane Phelan, 'Junior doctor gave "inappropriate prescriptions for multiple drugs" to young patients, whistleblower claims.' *Independent.ie*, 24 January 2022. https://www.independent. ie/irish-news/courts/junior-doctor-gave-inappropriate-prescriptions-for-multiple-drugs-to-young-patients-whistleblower-claims/41270705.html.

8 Sinead Kelleher. 'South Kerry CAMHS scandal revealed' *Independent.ie*, 23 December 2022. https://www.independent. ie/regionals/kerry/news/south-kerry-camhs-scandal-revealed/42238838.html#:~:text=The%20Maskey%20 Report%20-%20the%20result,in%20South%20Kerry%20 CAMHS%20services.

9 Martin Seligman. *Helplessness: On Depression, Development and Death*. New York: W. H. Freeman, 1975.

10 Mary Boyle and Lucy Johnstone. *A Straight Talking Introduction to the Power Threat Meaning Framework: An Alternative to Psychiatric Diagnosis*. Wales: PCCS Books, 2020.

11 Lucy Johnstone. *Psychiatric Diagnosis, revised second edition*. Wales: PCCS Books, 2022. 68.

Chapter Fifteen

1 Thich Nhat Hanh. *The Art of Living: Peace and Freedom in the Here and Now*. London: HarperOne, 2017.

Chapter Sixteen

1 J.R.R. Tolkien. *The Hobbit*. London: HarperCollins Children's Books, 2013.

2 David Foster Wallace. *This Is Water: Some Thoughts, Delivered on a Significant Occasion, about Living a Compassionate Life*. New York: Little, Brown and Company, 2009.

3 Sun Tzu. *The Art of War*. Singapore: Pax Librorum, 2009.

4 Helen McDonald. *Vesper Flights*. New York: Grove Press, 2020. 144.

5   Tony Bates. 'Nature can release us from mental turmoil: A year of living mindfully,' *Irish Times,* 18 June 2013.

6   Joseph Campbell. *The Power of Myth.* New York: Doubleday, 1988.

7   Thomas Merton. *The Inner Experience.* San Francisco: HarperOne, 2004. 5-7.

Chapter Seventeen

1   Nikita Gill. *These are the Words: Fearless Verse to Find your Voice.* New York: Macmillan, 2022.

2   Sigmund Freud, 'Remembering, repeating and working through', in vol 12 of *Standard Edition of the Complete Psychological Works of Sigmund Freud,* ed. and trans. James Strachey. London: Hogarth Press and Institute of Psychoanalysis, 1958. 152.

3   *Ibid.* 150.

4   D.W. Winnicott. 'Fear of Breakdown.' *International Review of Psychoanalysis.* 1 (1974): 106.

Chapter Eighteen

1   P. Bracken *et al.,* 'Psychiatry beyond the current paradigm.' *Cambridge University Press.* 2 January 2018. https://www.cambridge.org/core/journals/the-british-journal-of-psychiatry/article/psychiatry-beyond-the-current-paradigm/0EF061925997CA565C223DFE22BC3BEA.

2   *Ibid.* 150.

3   Bessel van der Kolk. 'Developmental trauma disorder: Toward a rational diagnosis for children with complex trauma histories.' *Psychiatric Annals,* 35. 5 (2005): 401–408.

4   Bruce Perry and Oprah Winfrey. *What Happened To You? Conversations on Trauma, Resilience and Healing.* London: Pan Macmillan, 2021. 112-115.

Chapter Nineteen

1   Joseph Campbell. 'Episode 1: The Hero's Adventure.' *The Power of Myth*. Distr. By PBS.

Epilogue

1   John Welwood. *Toward a Psychology of Awakening: Buddhism, Psychotherapy, and the Path of Personal and Spiritual Transformation*. Colorado: Shambhala Publications, 2002. 147.